Current MR Imaging of Breast Cancer

Editor

JESSICA W. T. LEUNG

MAGNETIC RESONANCE IMAGING CLINICS OF NORTH AMERICA

www.mri.theclinics.com

Consulting Editors
SURESH K. MUKHERJI
LYNNE S. STEINBACH

May 2018 • Volume 26 • Number 2

ELSEVIER

1600 John F. Kennedy Boulevard • Suite 1800 • Philadelphia, Pennsylvania, 19103-2899

http://www.mri.theclinics.com

MRI CLINICS OF NORTH AMERICA Volume 26, Number 2
May 2018 ISSN 1064-9689, ISBN 13: 978-0-323-58364-0

Editor: John Vassallo (j.vassallo@elsevier.com)
Developmental Editor: Meredith Madeira

Magnetic Resonance Imaging Clinics of North America (ISSN 1064-9689) is published quarterly by Elsevier Inc., 360 Park Avenue South, New York, NY 10010-1710. Months of issue are February, May, August, and November. Business and Editorial Offices: 1600 John F. Kennedy Blvd., Ste. 1800, Philadelphia, PA 19103-2899. Customer Service Office: 3251 Riverport Lane, Maryland Heights, MO 63043. Periodicals postage paid at New York, NY and additional mailing offices. Subscription prices are $395.00 per year (domestic individuals), $701.00 per year (domestic institutions), $100.00 per year (domestic students/residents), $437.00 per year (Canadian individuals), $913.00 per year (Canadian institutions), $545.00 per year (international individuals), $913.00 per year (international institutions), and $275.00 per year (international and Canadian students/residents). International air speed delivery is included in all *Clinics* subscription prices. All prices are subject to change without notice. **POSTMASTER:** Send address changes to *Magnetic Resonance Imaging Clinics*, Elsevier Health Sciences Division, Subscription Customer Service, 3251 Riverport Lane, Maryland Heights, MO 63043. Customer Service (orders, claims, online, change of address): Elsevier Health Sciences Division, Subscription **Customer Service, 3251 Riverport Lane, Maryland Heights, MO 63043. Tel:1-800-654-2452 (U.S. and Canada); 314-447-8871 (outside U.S. and Canada). Fax: 314-447-8029. E-mail: journalscustomer service-usa@elsevier.com (for print support); journalsonlinesupport-usa@elsevier.com (for online support).**

Reprints. For copies of 100 or more of articles in this publication, please contact the Commercial Reprints Department, Elsevier Inc., 360 Park Avenue South, New York, NY 10010-1710. Tel.: 212-633-3874; Fax: 212-633-3820; E-mail: reprints@elsevier.com.

Magnetic Resonance Imaging Clinics of North America is covered in the *RSNA Index of Imaging Literature, MEDLINE/PubMed (Index Medicus),* and *EMBASE/Excerpta Medica.*

Printed in the United States of America.

Contributors

CONSULTING EDITORS

SURESH K. MUKHERJI, MD, MBA, FACR
Professor and Chairman, Walter F. Patenge
Endowed Chair, Department of Radiology,
Michigan State University, Chief Medical
Officer and Director of Health Care Delivery,
Michigan State University Health Team,
East Lansing, Michigan

LYNNE S. STEINBACH, MD, FACR
Professor of Radiology and Orthopaedic
Surgery, Department of Radiology and
Biomedical Imaging, University of California,
San Francisco, San Francisco, California

EDITOR

JESSICA W.T. LEUNG, MD, FACR, FSBI
Section Chief, Breast Imaging, Professor,
Department of Diagnostic Radiology, Division
of Diagnostic Imaging, The University of Texas
MD Anderson Cancer Center, Houston, Texas

AUTHORS

BEATRIZ E. ADRADA, MD
Associate Professor, Department of Diagnostic
Radiology, Breast Imaging Section, The
University of Texas MD Anderson Cancer
Center, Houston, Texas

CATHERINE M. APPLETON, MD
Chief Breast Imaging Section, Associate
Professor, Mallinckrodt Institute of Radiology,
Washington University School of Medicine
in St. Louis, Saint Louis, Missouri

VIVIAN J. BEA, MD
Department of Breast Surgical Oncology,
The University of Texas MD Anderson Cancer
Center, Houston, Texas

ISABELLE BEDROSIAN, MD, FACS
Professor, Department of Breast Surgical
Oncology, The University of Texas MD
Anderson Cancer Center, Houston, Texas

WENDIE A. BERG, MD, PhD
Professor, Department of Radiology,
University of Pittsburgh School of Medicine,
Magee-Women's Hospital of UPMC,
Pittsburgh, Pennsylvania

ROSALIND P. CANDELARIA, MD
Assistant Professor, Department of Radiology,
The University of Texas MD Anderson Cancer
Center, Houston, Texas

KAITLIN M. CHRISTOPHERSON, MD
Resident Physician, Department of
Radiation Oncology, The University of Texas
MD Anderson Cancer Center, Houston,
Texas

ETHAN COHEN, MD
Assistant Professor, Department of Diagnostic
Radiology, Division of Diagnostic Imaging,
The University of Texas MD Anderson
Cancer Center, Houston, Texas

MATTHEW F. COVINGTON, MD
Assistant Professor, Mallinckrodt Institute of
Radiology, Washington University School of
Medicine in St. Louis, Saint Louis, Missouri

JESSICA H. HAYWARD, MD
Assistant Clinical Professor, Department of
Radiology and Biomedical Imaging, University
of California, San Francisco, San Francisco,
California

LAURA HEACOCK, MD
Assistant Professor of Radiology, NYU School of Medicine, NYU Laura and Isaac Perlmutter Cancer Center, New York, New York

SAMANTHA LYNN HELLER, MD, PhD
Assistant Professor of Radiology, NYU School of Medicine, NYU Laura and Isaac Perlmutter Cancer Center, New York, New York

MONICA L. HUANG, MD
Assistant Professor, Department of Radiology, The University of Texas MD Anderson Cancer Center, Houston, Texas

BONNIE N. JOE, MD, PhD
Professor in Residence and Chief of Breast Imaging, Department of Radiology and Biomedical Imaging, University of California, San Francisco, San Francisco, California

HUONG T. LE-PETROSS, MD
Professor, Department of Diagnostic Imaging, The University of Texas MD Anderson Cancer Center, Houston, Texas

JESSICA W.T. LEUNG, MD, FACR, FSBI
Section Chief, Breast Imaging, Professor, Department of Diagnostic Radiology, Division of Diagnostic Imaging, The University of Texas MD Anderson Cancer Center, Houston, Texas

JOHN LEWIN, MD
The Women's Imaging Center, Denver, Colorado

BORA LIM, MD
Assistant Professor, Department of Breast Medical Oncology, The University of Texas MD Anderson Cancer Center, Houston, Texas

SARAH R. MARTAINDALE, MD
Assistant Professor, Department of Diagnostic Radiology, Breast Imaging Section, The University of Texas MD Anderson Cancer Center, Houston, Texas

LINDA MOY, MD
Professor of Radiology, NYU School of Medicine, NYU Laura and Isaac Perlmutter Cancer Center, New York, New York

DEEPA NARAYANAN, MS
Program Director, SBIR Development Center, National Cancer Institute, Rockville, Maryland

BENJAMIN RABER, MD
Department of Surgery, Baylor University Medical Center, Dallas, Texas

AKSHARA S. RAGHAVENDRA, MD, MS
Department of Breast Medical Oncology, Division of Cancer Medicine, The University of Texas MD Anderson Cancer Center, Houston, Texas

GAIANE M. RAUCH, MD, PhD
Associate Professor, Department of Diagnostic Radiology, Abdominal and Breast Imaging Sections, Director of Molecular Breast Imaging, The University of Texas MD Anderson Cancer Center, Houston, Texas

KIMBERLY M. RAY, MD
Attending Radiologist, Kaiser Permanente, Oakland, California

LUMARIE SANTIAGO, MD
Associate Professor, Department of Radiology, The University of Texas MD Anderson Cancer Center, Houston, Texas

BENJAMIN D. SMITH, MD
Associate Professor, Department of Radiation Oncology, The University of Texas MD Anderson Cancer Center, Houston, Texas

DEBU TRIPATHY, MD
Department of Breast Medical Oncology, Division of Cancer Medicine, The University of Texas MD Anderson Cancer Center, Houston, Texas

CATHERINE A. YOUNG, MD, JD
Assistant Professor, Mallinckrodt Institute of Radiology, Washington University School of Medicine in St. Louis, Saint Louis, Missouri

Contents

Foreword: Breast MR Imaging   xi

Lynne S. Steinbach

Preface: Breast MR Imaging in Era of Value-Based Medicine   xiii

Jessica W.T. Leung

Breast MR Imaging: Atlas of Anatomy, Physiology, Pathophysiology, and Breast Imaging Reporting and Data Systems Lexicon   179

Sarah R. Martaindale

The latest edition of the Breast Imaging Reporting and Data Systems lexicon, copyrighted in 2013, contains several changes to the breast MR imaging section. Most changes were implemented to standardize descriptors across breast imaging modalities. New sections on special topics and implant evaluation are included. The authors review basic MR imaging breast anatomy and a detailed pictorial review of the Breast Imaging Reporting and Data Systems lexicon, including these new sections. Each section discusses which descriptors are more concerning for malignancy and information radiologists can use to better categorize findings as lower risk or benign.

Role of MR Imaging for the Locoregional Staging of Breast Cancer   191

Kimberly M. Ray, Jessica H. Hayward, and Bonnie N. Joe

Breast MR imaging has been shown to identify unsuspected sites of cancer in the ipsilateral breast in 16% of women with newly diagnosed breast cancer. Breast MR imaging identifies occult cancer in the contralateral breast in 3% to 5% of women. Early evidence suggests that the added value of MR imaging for staging may be attenuated in women who also undergo tomosynthesis, particularly those with nondense breasts. Breast MR imaging is complementary to ultrasound imaging in evaluating regional nodal basins. Ongoing prospective randomized clinical trials should clarify the impact of preoperative breast MR imaging on clinical outcomes.

Role of MR Imaging in Neoadjuvant Therapy Monitoring   207

Huong T. Le-Petross and Bora Lim

Neoadjuvant chemotherapy (NAC) has become an important treatment approach for stage II/III breast cancers to downsize tumor and enable breast-conserving surgery for patients who may otherwise undergo mastectomy. MR imaging has the potential to identify early response or disease progression, enabling potential modification to NAC regimens. Detection of size and morphologic changes is better appreciated with MR imaging than with other modalities and is different between molecular subtypes of breast cancer. The combination of DCE-MR imaging and DWI provides the highest sensitivity and specificity. Other new modalities such as FDG PET/MR imaging and molecular breast imaging are still undergoing research.

Problem-Solving MR Imaging for Equivocal Imaging Findings and Indeterminate Clinical Symptoms of the Breast   221

Ethan Cohen and Jessica W.T. Leung

Breast MR imaging is commonly used for high-risk screening and for assessing the extent of disease in patients with newly diagnosed breast cancer, but its utility for assessing suspicious symptoms and equivocal imaging findings is less widely accepted. The authors review the current literature and guidelines regarding the use of breast MR imaging for these indications. Overall, problem-solving breast MR imaging is best reserved for pathologic nipple discharge and sonographically occult architectural distortion with limited biopsy options. Further study is necessary to define the role of problem-solving MR imaging for calcifications, mammographic asymmetries, and surgical scarring.

MR Imaging–Guided Breast Interventions: Indications, Key Principles, and Imaging-Pathology Correlation

235

Lumarie Santiago, Rosalind P. Candelaria, and Monica L. Huang

MR imaging is now routinely performed for breast cancer screening and staging. For suspicious MR imaging–detected lesions that are mammographically and sonographically occult, MR imaging–guided breast interventions, including biopsy, clip placement, and preoperative needle localization, have been developed to permit accurate tissue diagnosis and aid in surgical planning. These procedures are safe, accurate, and effective when performed according to key principles, including proper patient selection, use of appropriate technique, adequate preprocedure preparation and postprocedure patient care, and postprocedure imaging-pathology correlation. Imaging-pathology correlation after MR imaging–guided biopsy is essential to confirm accurate sampling and guide development of a comprehensive management plan.

Developments in Breast Imaging: Update on New and Evolving MR Imaging and Molecular Imaging Techniques

247

Samantha Lynn Heller, Laura Heacock, and Linda Moy

This article reviews new developments in breast imaging. There is growing interest in creating a shorter, less expensive MR protocol with broader applicability. There is an increasing focus on and consideration for the additive impact that functional analyses of breast pathology have on identifying and characterizing lesions. These developments apply to MR imaging and molecular imaging. This article reviews evolving breast imaging techniques, with attention to strengths, weaknesses, and applications of these approaches. The authors aim to give the reader familiarity with the state of current developments in the field and to increase awareness of what to expect in breast imaging.

Comparison of Contrast-Enhanced Mammography and Contrast-Enhanced Breast MR Imaging

259

John Lewin

Contrast-enhanced mammography (CEM) is a contrast-enhanced modality for breast cancer detection that utilizes iodinated contrast and dual-energy imaging performed on a digital mammography unit with only slight modifications. It is approved by the US Food and Drug Administration, commercially available, and in routine clinical use at centers around the world. It has similar sensitivity and specificity to MR imaging and has advantages in terms of cost, patient acceptability, and examination time. MR imaging has some advantages compared with CEM, especially in its ability to image the complete axilla and the chest wall.

Use of Breast-Specific PET Scanners and Comparison with MR Imaging

265

Deepa Narayanan and Wendie A. Berg

This article discusses the role of breast-specific PET imaging of women with breast cancer, compares the clinical performance of positron emission mammography

(PEM) and MR imaging for current indications, and provides recommendations for when women should undergo PEM instead of breast MR imaging.

Comparison of Breast MR Imaging with Molecular Breast Imaging in Breast Cancer Screening, Diagnosis, Staging, and Treatment Response Evaluation   273

Gaiane M. Rauch and Beatriz E. Adrada

Breast MR imaging and molecular breast imaging (MBI) are functional imaging modalities that can be used to noninvasively evaluate the pathophysiology and biology of breast cancer. In the era of personalized medicine, these imaging techniques give clinicians insight into cancer pathobiology and allows them to individualize treatment regimens. Breast MR imaging has gained acceptance for breast cancer evaluation; work is ongoing on validation of MBI for breast cancer evaluation. This article discusses clinical applications of breast MR imaging and MBI and compares the performance of these techniques in breast cancer screening, diagnosis, staging, and treatment response evaluation.

How Does MR Imaging Help Care for My Breast Cancer Patient? Perspective of a Surgical Oncologist   281

Benjamin Raber, Vivian J. Bea, and Isabelle Bedrosian

MR imaging is now readily available for surgeons to incorporate into their practice, thus, begging the question, is this new modality clinically useful? The current literature and expert opinion are reviewed concerning the implementation of breast MR imaging to clinical management of breast cancer. Although breast MR imaging is acknowledged to be highly sensitive in the detection of breast cancer, its routine application to surgical practice remains controversial because these gains in sensitivity have not been demonstrated to translate into improved long-term patient outcomes. Current clinical trials and the future of breast MR imaging are also discussed.

How Does MR Imaging Help Care for the Breast Cancer Patient? Perspective of a Medical Oncologist   289

Akshara S. Raghavendra and Debu Tripathy

Although traditional assessment with clinical examination, mammogram, and ultrasound is generally accepted for detection and staging of breast cancer, MR imaging is commonly used to detect occult cancers in the breast and regional nodes in the early stage and to determine the extent of disease in patients with metastatic disease. Several studies have shown a variety of uses for MR imaging in the staging of breast cancer and assessment of treatment response in the neoadjuvant (preoperative) setting. This article reviews the impact of MR imaging in different settings on medical oncology decision making in patients with breast cancer.

How Does MR Imaging Help Care for My Breast Cancer Patient? Perspective of a Radiation Oncologist   295

Kaitlin M. Christopherson and Benjamin D. Smith

Radiation therapy is used in many cases of both early and late breast cancer. The authors examine the role of MR imaging as it pertains to radiotherapy planning and treatment approaches for patients with breast cancer. MR imaging can assist the radiation oncologist in determining the best radiation approach and in creating treatment planning volumes. MR imaging may be useful in the setting of accelerated partial breast irradiation. Radiation oncologists should attend to MR breast images, when obtained, to ensure that these imaging findings are taken into consideration when developing a radiation therapy plan.

American College of Radiology Accreditation, Performance Metrics, Reimbursement, and Economic Considerations in Breast MR Imaging   303

Matthew F. Covington, Catherine A. Young, and Catherine M. Appleton

Accreditation through the American College of Radiology (ACR) Breast Magnetic Resonance Imaging Accreditation Program is necessary to qualify for reimbursement from Medicare and many private insurers and provides facilities with peer review on image acquisition and clinical quality. Adherence to ACR quality control and technical practice parameter guidelines for breast MR imaging and performance of a medical outcomes audit program will maintain high-quality imaging and facilitate accreditation. Economic factors likely to influence the practice of breast MR imaging include cost-effectiveness, competition with lower-cost breast-imaging modalities, and price transparency, all of which may lower the cost of MR imaging and allow for greater utilization.

MAGNETIC RESONANCE IMAGING CLINICS OF NORTH AMERICA

FORTHCOMING ISSUES

August 2018
MR Imaging of the Pancreas
Kumar Sandrasegaran and Dushyant V. Sahani, *Editors*

November 2018
Advanced MSK Imaging
Roberto Domingues and Flavia Costa, *Editors*

February 2019
MR Imaging of the Genitourinary System
Ersan Altun, *Editor*

RECENT ISSUES

February 2018
State-of-the-Art Imaging of Head and Neck Tumors
Girish M. Fatterpekar, *Editor*

November 2017
Update on Imaging Contrast Agents
Carlos A. Zamora and Mauricio Castillo, *Editors*

August 2017
Gynecologic Imaging
Katherine E. Maturen, *Editor*

ISSUE OF RELATED INTEREST

Radiologic Clinics of North America, May 2017 (Vol. 55, No. 3)
Breast Imaging
Sarah M. Friedewald, *Editor*
Available at: www.radiologic.theclinics.com

VISIT THE CLINICS ONLINE!
Access your subscription at:
www.theclinics.com

PROGRAM OBJECTIVE

The goal of *Magnetic Resonance Imaging Clinics of North America* is to keep practicing physicians up to date with current clinical practice by providing timely articles reviewing the state of the art in patient care.

TARGET AUDIENCE

All practicing physicians and healthcare professionals who provide patient care utilizing findings from Magnetic Resonance Imaging.

LEARNING OBJECTIVES

Upon completion of this activity, participants will be able to:
1. Review new and evolving developments in breast Imaging interventions and screening
2. Discuss perspectives of MRI care for breast cancer patients
3. Recognize ACR accreditation, Performance Metrics, Reimbursement, and Economic Considerations in Breast MRI

ACCREDITATION

The Elsevier Office of Continuing Medical Education (EOCME) is accredited by the Accreditation Council for Continuing Medical Education (ACCME) to provide continuing medical education for physicians.

The EOCME designates this enduring material for a maximum of 15 *AMA PRA Category 1 Credit*(s)™. Physicians should claim only the credit commensurate with the extent of their participation in the activity.

All other healthcare professionals requesting continuing education credit for this enduring material will be issued a certificate of participation.

DISCLOSURE OF CONFLICTS OF INTEREST

The EOCME assesses conflict of interest with its instructors, faculty, planners, and other individuals who are in a position to control the content of CME activities. All relevant conflicts of interest that are identified are thoroughly vetted by EOCME for fair balance, scientific objectivity, and patient care recommendations. EOCME is committed to providing its learners with CME activities that promote improvements or quality in healthcare and not a specific proprietary business or a commercial interest.

The planning committee, staff, authors and editors listed below have identified no financial relationships or relationships to products or devices they or their spouse/life partner have with commercial interest related to the content of this CME activity:

Beatriz E. Adrada, MD; Catherine M. Appleton, MD; Vivian J. Bea, MD; Isabelle Bedrosian, MD, FACS; Wendie A. Berg, MD, PhD; Rosalind P. Candelaria, MD; Kaitlin M. Christopherson, MD; Ethan Cohen, MD; Matthew F. Covington, MD; Jessica H. Hayward, MD; Laura Heacock, MD; Samantha Lynn Heller, MD, PhD; Monica L. Huang, MD; Bonnie N. Joe, MD, PhD; Alison Kemp; Huong T. Le-Petross, MD; Jessica W.T. Leung, MD, FACR, FSBI; John Lewin, MD; Bora Lim, MD; Sarah R. Martaindale, MD; Linda Moy, MD; Deepa Narayanan, MS; Benjamin Raber, MD; Akshara S. Raghavendra, MD, MS; Gaiane M. Rauch, MD, PhD; Kimberly M. Ray, MD; Lumarie Santiago, MD; Benjamin D. Smith, MD; Lynne S. Steinbach, MD, FACR; Karthik Subramaniam; Debu Tripathy, MD; John Vassallo; Catherine A.Young, MD, JD.

UNAPPROVED/OFF-LABEL USE DISCLOSURE

The EOCME requires CME faculty to disclose to the participants:
1. When products or procedures being discussed are off-label, unlabelled, experimental, and/or investigational (not US Food and Drug Administration [FDA] approved); and
2. Any limitations on the information presented, such as data that are preliminary or that represent ongoing research, interim analyses, and/or unsupported opinions. Faculty may discuss information about pharmaceutical agents that is outside of FDA-approved labelling. This information is intended solely for CME and is not intended to promote off-label use of these medications. If you have any questions, contact the medical affairs department of the manufacturer for the most recent prescribing information.

TO ENROLL

To enroll in the *Magnetic Resonance Imaging Clinics of North America* Continuing Medical Education program, call customer service at 1-800-654-2452 or sign up online at http://www.theclinics.com/home/cme. The CME program is available to subscribers for an additional annual fee of USD 260.

METHOD OF PARTICIPATION

In order to claim credit, participants must complete the following:
1. Complete enrolment as indicated above.
2. Read the activity.
3. Complete the CME Test and Evaluation. Participants must achieve a score of 70% on the test. All CME Tests and Evaluations must be completed online.

CME INQUIRIES/SPECIAL NEEDS

For all CME inquiries or special needs, please contact elsevierCME@elsevier.com.

Foreword
Breast MR Imaging

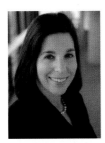

Lynne S. Steinbach, MD, FACR
Consulting Editor

We are excited to present this new issue on breast MR imaging. It contains many important and timely topics that cover this rapidly changing field. This will be a valuable updated resource for all breast imagers as well as those who treat breast cancer.

The series editor, Jessica Leung, MD, is a world-renowned breast imager who is currently the Chief of Breast Imaging at the University of Texas MD Anderson Cancer Center in Houston. She has assembled a distinguished group of breast imagers and treatment specialists from MD Anderson and other top institutions to contribute updates on these important areas.

Sarah Martaindale, MD from MD Anderson presents a fundamental article that provides a refresher of the essential anatomy, physiology, and pathophysiology with the latest edition of the MR imaging BI-RADs lexicon that brings consistency to the descriptors used across the BI-RADS lexicon and eliminates underutilized or confusing terminology.

Monitoring of neoadjuvant therapy with MR imaging is covered by MD Anderson physicians Huong T. Le Petross, MD and Bora Lim, MD. One of their conclusions is that a combination of dynamic contrast-enhanced MR imaging and diffusion-weighted imaging provides better technique and promising tools for predicting response to neoadjuvant therapy, enabling early modification to therapy.

MR imaging–guided breast interventions: indications, key principles, and imaging-pathology correlation, is discussed by radiologists Lumarie Santiago, MD, Rosalind P. Candelaria, MD, and Monica L. Huang, MD from MD Anderson. They emphasize that imaging-pathologic correlation after MR imaging–guided biopsy is essential to confirm accurate sampling and to guide creation of a multidisciplinary management plan.

An update on new and evolving MR imaging and molecular imaging techniques is provided by Samantha Lynn Heller, MD, PhD, Laura Heacock, MD, and Linda Moy, MD from New York University Medical Center. This covers the latest on a variety of MR sequences and molecular imaging, including PET/MR. They also explore the use of protocols that shorten the MR examination time.

American College of Radiology accreditation, performance metrics, reimbursement, and economic considerations in Breast MR imaging is comprehensively covered by Matthew F. Covington, MD from Mayo Clinic Scottsdale and Catherine A. Young, MD, JD and Catherine M. Appleton, MD from Mallinckrodt Institute of Radiology in St Louis. They provide critical operational and financial information for any radiologist or group that is reading breast studies.

Kimberly Ray, MD, Jessica Hayward, MD, and Bonnie Joe, MD, PhD at University of California San Francisco compare MR imaging with ultrasound and tomosynthesis regarding the extent of breast disease. There is also a special focus on nodal assessment. Some of the take-home points include the fact that MR imaging can be used preoperatively to detect unsuspected sites in the contralateral breast and can be useful for nodal evaluation.

A useful guide to problem-solving using MR imaging for equivocal imaging findings and indeterminate clinical symptoms of the breast is included. MD Anderson radiologists Ethan Cohen, MD and Jessica Leung, MD emphasize that problem-solving strongly depends on high-quality technique and appropriate case selection.

Magn Reson Imaging Clin N Am 26 (2018) xi–xii
https://doi.org/10.1016/j.mric.2018.02.002
1064-9689/18/© 2018 Published by Elsevier Inc.

John Lewin, MD from the Women's Imaging Center in Denver, Colorado compares contrast-enhanced mammography and contrast-enhanced breast MR imaging. Among other interesting observations are that contrast-enhanced mammography sensitivity is similar to that of MR imaging, and the specificity of contrast-enhanced mammography is superior to MR imaging.

Another area that is covered compares breast MR imaging with molecular breast imaging (MBI). It is coauthored by Gaiane Ruch, MD, PhD and Beatriz Adrada, MD from MD Anderson. The advantages and disadvantages of each type of imaging are mentioned, including the lack of radiation with MR imaging and the greater specificity, lower cost, and absence of nephrotoxicity, limitations to body weight, and claustrophobia with MBI.

A comparison of positron emission mammography (PEM) with MR imaging is provided by Deepa Narayanan, MS and Wendie Berg, MD, PhD from the National Cancer Institute and the University of Pittsburgh, respectively. PEM is similar in sensitivity and more specific than MR imaging. It is useful where breast MR imaging is contraindicated.

Surgical oncologists, Benjamin Raber, MD from Baylor University Medical Center in Houston, as well as Vivian Bea, MD and Isabelle Bedrosian, MD from MD Anderson provide a surgeon's perspective on the use of breast MR imaging for their patients. While pointing out that improved local staging alters surgical therapy in a substantial number of patients with breast cancer, these authors also discuss some disadvantages of MR imaging, including low specificity, increased cost, and negative biopsy rate as well as increased patient anxiety associated with the increased biopsy rate. They suggest the particular patient populations that would benefit from breast MR imaging.

Two medical oncologists, Akshara Raghavendra, MD, MS and Debu Tripathy, MD, from MD Anderson also give their perspective on the role of MR imaging for the patient with breast cancer. They discuss the various roles of MR imaging in conjunction with clinical examination, mammography, and ultrasound.

Last but not least, Kaitlin Christopherson, MD and Benjamin Smith, MD, who are radiation oncologists at MD Anderson, give their review of the role of MR imaging of the breast for their particular treatment. MR imaging can determine who would be eligible for accelerated partial breast irradiation and can accurately and consistently delineate target volume preoperatively. Late sequelae of radiation is also nicely evaluated with MR imaging.

In summary, Dr Leung has assembled an impressive group of authorities in the world of breast cancer imaging and treatment to discuss timely topics on the diagnosis and treatment of breast cancer. We congratulate all of the authors on their excellent contributions.

Lynne S. Steinbach, MD, FACR
Department of Radiology and
Biomedical Imaging
University of California San Francisco
505 Parnassus
San Francisco, CA 9413-0628, USA

E-mail address:
lynne.steinbach@ucsf.edu

Preface

Breast MR Imaging in Era of Value-Based Medicine

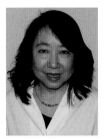

Jessica W.T. Leung, MD, FACR, FSBI

Editor

We live in an era of value-based medicine. While breast cancer remains the most commonly diagnosed nonskin cancer and a major cause of mortality and morbidity worldwide, affecting not only the lives of patients but also those of their families and friends, it is increasingly important that we utilize our finite resources in a cost-efficient and (whenever possible) evidence-based manner. This issue of *Magnetic Resonance Imaging Clinics of North America* has been constructed with these guiding thoughts.

This publication begins with an overview of breast MR imaging BI-RADS, the shared lexicon and approach we use for breast MR imaging interpretation and patient management. Subsequent articles focus on generally accepted (albeit controversial in specifics) breast MR imaging indications: defining extent of disease, neoadjuvant therapy monitoring, and problem-solving. These articles are followed by a practical and clinically important discussion on the "nuts and bolts" of MR imaging–guided breast biopsy, with emphasis on imaging-pathology concordance. As MR imaging technology continues to evolve, the next article discusses some of the most clinically pertinent current developments, including diffusion techniques and abbreviated MR imaging protocols.

It is important to remember that MR imaging does not stand alone as an imaging test. When compared with the other conventional breast imaging modalities of mammography and ultrasound, breast MR imaging is unique in that it affords functional (in addition to structural) information. How does it compare with the other functional breast imaging tests currently available for clinical use? The articles on contrast-enhanced mammography, breast-specific PET, and molecular breast imaging provide insight.

The success of MR imaging in clinical practice is highly dependent on its contributions to direct patient care. To this end, this issue highlights perspectives on breast MR imaging from our clinical colleagues (surgeons, medical oncologists, and radiation oncologists), without whom our imaging tests would be much less meaningful.

As a final reminder that we live in an era of value-based medicine, the issue concludes with an article on breast MR imaging accreditation, performance metrics, reimbursement, and other economic considerations. Increasingly, and ever so importantly, we must demonstrate our contributions to patient

Magn Reson Imaging Clin N Am 26 (2018) xiii–xiv
https://doi.org/10.1016/j.mric.2018.02.001
1064-9689/18/

care as radiologists and ensure that this care is safe, appropriate, timely, patient-centric, and cost-effective.

I thank all the authors for generously sharing their knowledge and contributing to this issue. I am indebted to the wonderful staff at the *Clinics* division of Elsevier in realizing this publication, with special thanks to Meredith Madeira for her unrelenting and invaluable support and to John Vassallo for his vision in the *Magnetic Resonance Imaging Clinics of North America* series over many years. I dedicate this issue to my family for their unconditional support in all things I do, with special dedication to my father and role model,

Pui Chee Leung, who epitomizes scholarly pursuits even in the most challenging of times.

Jessica W.T. Leung, MD, FACR, FSBI
Department of Diagnostic Radiology
Division of Diagnostic Imaging
The University of Texas
MD Anderson Cancer Center
1155 Pressler Street
Unit 1350, CPB5.3201
Houston, TX 77030, USA

E-mail address:
JWLeung@mdanderson.org

Breast MR Imaging
Atlas of Anatomy, Physiology, Pathophysiology, and Breast Imaging Reporting and Data Systems Lexicon

Sarah R. Martaindale, MD

KEYWORDS

- Breast MR Imaging • BI-RADS • Anatomy • Atlas

KEY POINTS

- The latest edition of the MR imaging Breast Imaging Reporting and Data Systems lexicon brings consistency to the descriptors used across the lexicon and eliminates underused or confusing terminology.
- A more cohesive set of descriptors aids in lesion management and ultimately improves patient care by facilitating communication between radiologists and referring physicians.
- A new section on breast MR imaging implant evaluation assists radiologists in identifying key signs of implant rupture and effectively communicating those findings to surgeons.

INTRODUCTION

In 1993, the first edition of the Breast Imaging Reporting and Data System (BI-RADS) was released with the goal of standardizing mammography reporting and interpretation.[1] Ten years later in 2003, MR imaging was added to the fourth edition of the BI-RADS lexicon to provide consistency in communication of findings across modalities.[2] With the fifth edition of the American College of Radiology BI-RADS in 2013 came some important changes to the breast MR imaging lexicon as well as the mammography and breast ultrasound imaging lexicons. Several of these changes worked to unify terms across breast imaging modalities and eliminate confusing or underused terms.[3]

ANATOMY

Knowledge of the breast anatomy can assist with providing helpful descriptions and properly relaying important information, particularly for surgical planning. Components of the breast include the skin, superficial fascia, deep fascia, breast parenchyma, and the nipple–areola complex. The breast parenchyma is composed of a glandular epithelium, fibrous stroma, and fat. The glandular epithelium is composed of 15 to 20 lobes, which are in turn composed of lobules or terminal ductules, the milk-producing glands. Each breast lobe leads to a duct that widens to form a lactiferous sinus under the nipple–areolar complex, which then exits the nipple. The fibrous stroma, commonly referred to as Cooper's ligaments, consists of bands of connective tissue that traverse the breast and insert into the dermis. The breast parenchyma is enclosed by the superficial fascia, which lies just beneath the skin, and the deep fascia, which envelops the pectoralis major muscle. Overlying the superficial fascia is the skin.[4] **Fig. 1** illustrates these basic anatomic structures of the breast as seen on a typical sagittal MR imaging sequence.

Disclosure Statement: The author has nothing to disclose.
Department of Diagnostic Radiology, Breast Imaging Section, The University of Texas MD Anderson Cancer Center, 1515 Holcombe Boulevard, Unit 1350, Houston, TX 77030, USA
E-mail address: smartaindale@mdanderson.org

Magn Reson Imaging Clin N Am 26 (2018) 179–190
https://doi.org/10.1016/j.mric.2017.12.001

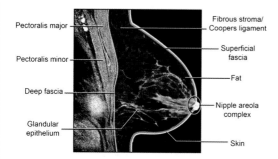

Fig. 1. Sagittal delayed postcontrast image demonstrating major anatomic components of the breast.

THE MR IMAGING BREAST IMAGING REPORTING AND DATA SYSTEMS LEXICON

The lexicon is divided into sections dedicated to detailing each component of a breast MR imaging examination. These sections begin with general breast parenchyma characteristics, such as the amount of fibroglandular tissue and the degree of background parenchymal enhancement (BPE). Next, we review multiple types of lesion findings, including focus, mass, nonmass enhancement, multiple benign entities, associated findings of importance when evaluating a malignancy, enhancement kinetics, and, last, implant evaluation.

BREAST TISSUE

The addition of a descriptor of the amount of fibroglandular tissue within the breast, similar to that long used for mammography, is new for this edition of the BI-RADS lexicon. On MR imaging, the amount of fibroglandular tissue should be assessed on a T1-weighted image using 1 of 4 descriptors: almost entirely fat, scattered fibroglandular tissue, heterogeneous fibroglandular tissue, or extreme fibroglandular tissue (Fig. 2).

Also new is the addition of a statement on the BPE, which is defined based on the enhancement of the patient's fibroglandular tissue on the first postcontrast sequence. Descriptor categories include minimal, mild, moderate, or marked. Important to note is that the term "multiple foci" has been removed from the lexicon with the understanding that this represents a pattern of background enhancement. The distinction between the amount of fibroglandular tissue and BPE is important because the degree of BPE is not necessarily related to the amount of breast tissue (Fig. 3). The degree of BPE is largely influenced by hormonal factors related to the menstrual cycle and it is generally recommended that nonurgent (screening or follow-up) breast MR imaging be scheduled during days 7 to 15 (week 2) of the menstrual cycle to minimize these effects.[5] Although previously theorized that BPE may limit the ability of MR imaging to adequately detect malignancy, that has not been found to be the case. Studies evaluating the effects of BPE on the accuracy of breast MR imaging have shown that an increased amount of BPE may lead to an increased recall rate, but does not decrease the cancer detection rate.[6,7]

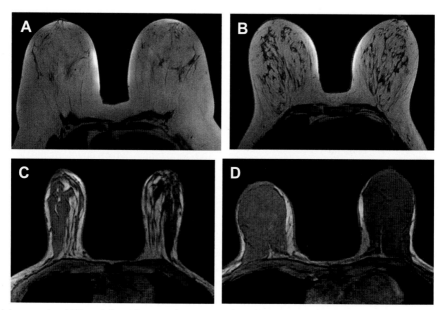

Fig. 2. Axial precontrast T1-weighted images show examples of almost entirely fat (A), scattered fibroglandular tissue (B), heterogeneous fibroglandular tissue (C), and extreme fibroglandular tissue (D).

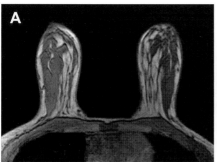
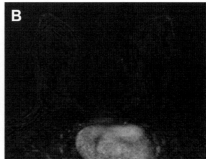

Fig. 3. Axial precontrast T1-weighted (*A*) and subtraction image (*B*) of the same patient at the same level demonstrating heterogeneous fibroglandular tissue with minimal background parenchymal enhancement.

Included in the discussion of BPE is a descriptor for symmetric versus asymmetric enhancement (**Fig. 4**). Symmetric enhancement is benign bilateral, "mirror image" enhancement that often appears in the upper outer quadrants and the inferior breasts. In prior versions of the BI-RADS lexicon, this was referred to as "sheets of enhancement," a term now removed from the lexicon. Asymmetric enhancement may be benign or malignant and describes enhancement that is more prominent in 1 breast. Clinical history of prior radiation therapy for breast cancer can explain asymmetric BPE, because the irradiated breast will have less enhancement than the nonirradiated breast.

BREAST LESIONS

Next, we discuss the updated terms for findings within the breast. Many of the terminology changes in this section were enacted to bring more consistency in reporting between breast MR imaging and other modalities. This update aids in clear communication of findings between radiologists as well as the referring clinicians. Applying the appropriate descriptors can also assist the radiologist with decision making for each lesion, because certain terms carry a higher risk of malignancy and may guide toward a biopsy or follow-up.

Focus

What is the difference between a focus and a mass? According to the American College of Radiology BI-RADS lexicon, a focus is punctate enhancement that is too small to characterize and has no precontrast correlate (**Fig. 5**). In prior versions, a size criterion of less than 5 mm was set, but the current version sets no strict size criteria because some masses are now identifiable and describable at this size with improved MR imaging technology resulting in better resolution. Now the difference between a focus and a mass is determined by the interpreting radiologist. Features that may assist with differentiating a benign focus from a malignant one are compared in **Table 1**. Most foci are benign, related to hormonal stimulation or underlying benign lesions (fibrocystic changes, fibroadenoma, cyst), but can rarely represent an early malignancy.[8,9] A recent study specifically assessed how frequently foci identified on MR imaging were malignant using follow-up MR imaging over a 5-year period and found that about 97% of foci identified were stable or disappeared on follow-up, and were therefore benign. The malignant foci were identified by biopsy after an increase in size on MR imaging and/or suspicious change in characteristics of the focus in only 2.9% of cases.[10]

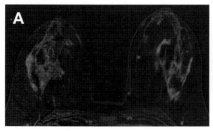
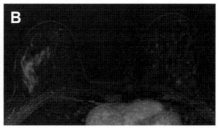

Fig. 4. Axial subtraction images demonstrating symmetric background parenchymal enhancement (BPE) (*A*) and asymmetric BPE (*B*).

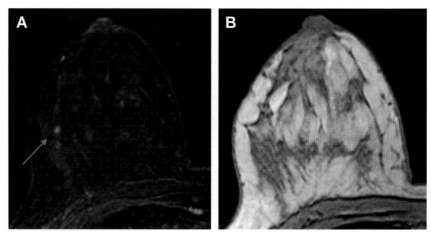

Fig. 5. Example of a focus denoted by a *red arrow* on axial subtraction image (*A*) with no correlate on axial pre-contrast T1-weighted image (*B*).

Mass

Contrasting with a focus, a mass is large enough to be described and is a space-occupying lesion that may present with a variety of shapes, margins, and internal enhancement characteristics. Terms available to describe the shape include oval, round, and irregular (**Fig. 6**). Of note, the term oval now encompasses the former term lobulated, which was removed from the current lexicon. Margins may be described as circumscribed (which was previously called "smooth"), irregular, or spiculated (**Fig. 7**). To describe a mass as having circumscribed margins, the entire mass must be circumscribed. If any part of the mass has irregular or spiculated margin, that descriptor should be used, because those terms convey a higher level of suspicion. Studies evaluating the positive predictive value of lesion characteristics on MR imaging have found a spiculated margin to have the highest likelihood of malignancy compared with other shape and margin descriptors.[11–13] Although the term indistinct is not included in this version of the lexicon, the term is under consideration for an upcoming edition. Descriptors of internal mass enhancement include homogeneous, heterogeneous, rim enhancement, and dark internal septations (**Fig. 8**). Rim enhancement is usually a malignant feature compared with other enhancement descriptors,[11–13] but cysts and fat necrosis should first be excluded using other sequences and/or available mammograms. The presence of dark internal septations suggests a fibroadenoma if other features support benignity. The terms "central enhancement" and "enhancing internal septations" have been removed owing to a lack of clinical relevance.

Nonmass Enhancement

Our next finding for discussion is nonmass enhancement (previously called nonmass-like enhancement). This describes enhancement that is discrete from the BPE but is neither a focus nor a mass. One important component of the description of nonmass enhancement is the distribution. Options to describe the distribution include focal, linear, segmental, regional, multiple regions, and diffuse (**Fig. 9**). Focal distribution is enhancement within a single duct and involving less than a quadrant. Linear distribution is within a single or branching line, and includes enhancement previously described as "ductal," which has been eliminated from the lexicon. Segmental distribution is triangular or conical-shaped, with the apex oriented toward the nipple. Regional distribution describes enhancement, which involves at least a quadrant, is geographic, and has no convex margins. Multiple regions describe the same appearance as regional distribution but at least 2 broad areas separated by normal tissue. Diffuse distribution is widely scattered and evenly distributed throughout the tissue. Diffuse distribution is

Table 1 Features of a focus	
Malignant Features	**Benign Features**
Not bright on T2-weighted imaging	Bright on T2-weighted imaging
No fatty hilum	Fatty hilum
Washout kinetics	Persistent kinetics
Larger or new since prior examination	Stable since prior examination

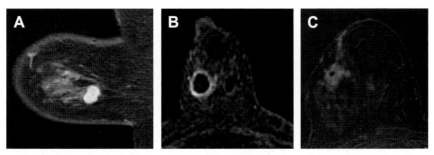

Fig. 6. (A) Sagittal delayed postcontrast fat saturated T1-weighted image demonstrates an oval mass. Axial subtraction images demonstrate a round mass (B) and an irregular mass (C).

generally benign whereas segmental or linear distribution has a higher risk of malignancy.[11,14-17]

The next component of nonmass enhancement description is the pattern of enhancement. Nonmass enhancement patterns of enhancement include homogeneous, heterogeneous, clumped, and clustered ring (Fig. 10). Clumped enhancement is a suspicious finding[11,14,15] and has previously been described as a cobblestone or string of pearls appearance. Clustered ring enhancement is a new term and describes multiple thin rings of enhancement. Clustered ring enhancement is a suspicious finding, although the differential diagnosis includes benign entities such as duct ectasia, fibrocystic change, and papilloma in addition to malignancy (ductal carcinoma in situ and invasive carcinoma). Studies have identified a positive predictive value for malignancy with clustered ring enhancement from 77% to 100%.[15-17] Of note, the terms "reticular" and "dendritic" have been eliminated from the lexicon owing to underuse.

Benign and Nonenhancing Findings

Also new for this edition is a section on special topics. These entities are all benign, and the inclusion of this section largely serves to assist readers in identifying and separating these relatively common findings from ones that require additional evaluation or biopsy. Specifically discussed are intramammary lymph nodes, skin lesions, and nonenhancing findings. Intramammary lymph nodes are a common benign mammographic finding, so it should come as no surprise that they would be commonly identified on MR imaging as well. Intramammary lymph nodes are circumscribed, reniform, homogeneously enhancing masses with hilar fat; are usually less than 1 cm in size; and are most commonly located in the upper outer quadrant. A close association with a vessel is a helpful feature. Skin lesions such as keloids, sebaceous cysts, postsurgical scar, and dermatitis can also be identified as enhancing findings within the skin, and are benign. Several nonenhancing findings are also described (Fig. 11). Duct ectasia can be identified by the high signal intensity within the ducts on precontrast T1-weighted images. Cysts may appear as signal voids on subtraction images, but will have associated high intensity T2-weighted signal. Varying degrees of susceptibility artifact can be seen in association with biopsy marker clips and other metallic

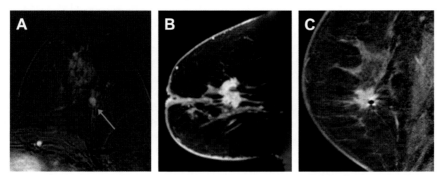

Fig. 7. Axial subtraction image demonstrates a mass with circumscribed margin, denoted by a red arrow (A). Sagittal postcontrast fat-saturated T1-weighted images demonstrate mass with irregular margin (B) and a mass with spiculated margin (C).

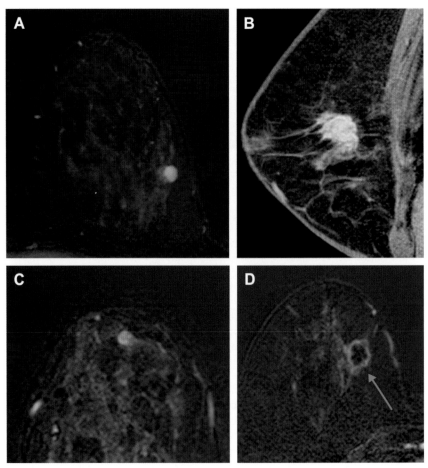

Fig. 8. Axial subtraction image of an oval mass with homogeneous enhancement (*A*). Sagittal postcontrast fat-saturated T1-weighted image of an irregular mass with heterogeneous enhancement (*B*). Axial subtraction images of an oval mass with dark internal septations (*C*) and a round mass with rim enhancement denoted by the *red arrow* (*D*).

foreign bodies, and correlation with mammography can assist in identifying the source of susceptibility artifacts. Knowing the patient's treatment history is important in correctly identifying skin and trabecular thickening as benign postradiation changes. Clinical history can also assist with correctly identifying nonenhancing architectural distortion from postbiopsy or post-surgical changes as well as postoperative collections. Sequences obtained without and with fat suppression can assist in accurately identifying benign, fat-containing lesions such as lymph nodes, fat necrosis, hamartoma (**Fig. 12**), and postoperative collections with fat.

Associated Features

There are several associated features that can be identified on MR imaging examinations that increase suspicion for breast cancer in undiagnosed patients and can alter staging and surgical management in those patients who have already been diagnosed with breast cancer. Just as on mammography, nipple retraction can be identified on MR imaging. Nipple invasion by a mass is an important finding and can alter the surgical options available to the patient. Direct skin invasion and pectoralis muscle or chest wall invasion should be described if present to allow for appropriate treatment planning. Sometimes these findings can be quite subtle on other imaging modalities or not recognized at all without the use of MR imaging. Although we have seen examples of benign skin thickening associated with postradiation changes, skin thickening can also be seen as an associated feature of breast malignancy. An important differentiating factor is concurrent enhancement in the area of skin thickening. Suspicious axillary lymphadenopathy will demonstrate effacement of the fatty hilum and a heterogeneous

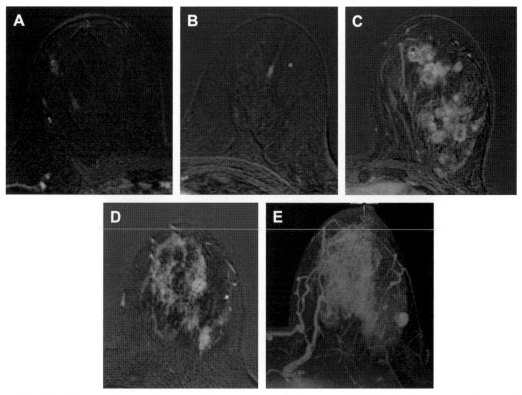

Fig. 9. Axial subtraction images demonstrate focal nonmass enhancement (NME) (*A*), linear NME (*B*), segmental NME (*C*), and regional NME (*D*). Axially oriented maximum intensity projection image demonstrates a mass and diffuse NME (*E*).

enhancement pattern compared with the homogeneous pattern seen with benign/normal lymph nodes. **Fig. 13** provides examples of several of these associated features.

KINETIC CURVE ASSESSMENT

Once the breast lesions of interest have been identified, enhancement kinetics characteristics should be evaluated and reported for each finding.

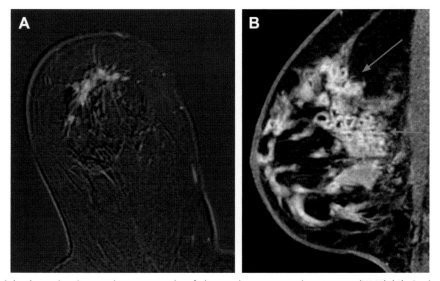

Fig. 10. Axial subtraction image shows example of clumped nonmass enhancement (NME) (*A*). Sagittal delayed postcontrast T1-weighted image demonstrates clustered ring NME, annotated by the *red arrows* (*B*).

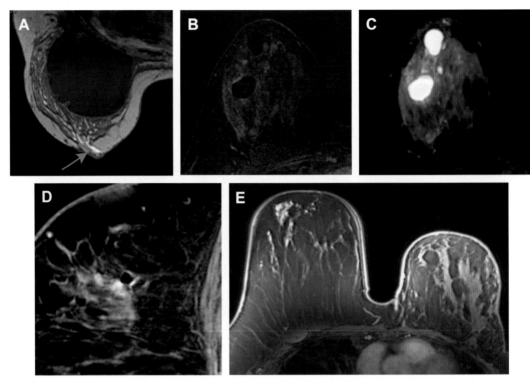

Fig. 11. Nonenhancing findings. Axial precontrast T1-weighted image with *red arrow* denotating the high signal intensity within multiple ducts, consistent with duct ectasia (*A*). Axial subtraction image and fat-saturated T2-weighted images from the same patient demonstrate oval nonenhancing signal voids (*B*) with high signal intensity (*C*) on T2-weighted images, consistent with cysts. Sagittal delayed postcontrast fat-saturated image with susceptibility artifact from biopsy marker clip (*D*). Axial postcontrast fat-saturated image demonstrating nonenhancing left breast skin thickening and trabecular thickening in a patient with history of left breast cancer and treatment changes from radiation therapy (*E*).

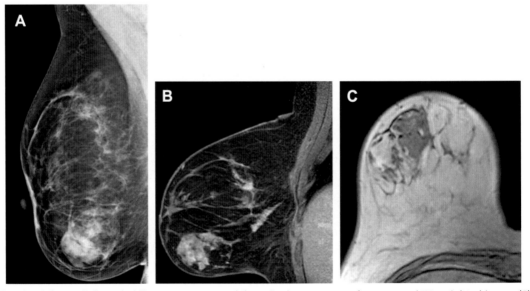

Fig. 12. Right mediolateral oblique mammogram (*A*), sagittal postcontrast fat-saturated T1-weighted image (*B*) and axial precontrast non–fat-saturated image (*C*) of an oval fat containing mass, consistent with hamartoma.

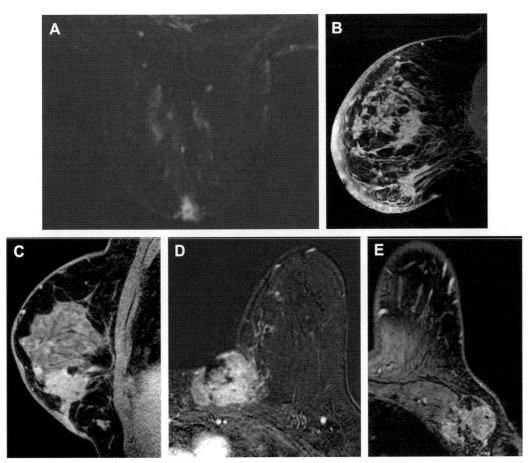

Fig. 13. Associated features. Axial subtraction image demonstrates nipple invasion by malignancy (*A*). Axial post-contrast fat-saturated image with diffuse skin and trabecular thickening (*B*) that enhances, making this a suspicious feature compared with the nonenhancing skin and trabecular thickening associated with radiation therapy shown in **Fig. 11**. Sagittal postcontrast fat saturated image with direct skin invasion by the breast malignancy (*C*). Axial subtraction image demonstrating pectoralis major and skin invasion by the malignancy (*D*). Axial subtraction image showing matted axillary lymphadenopathy in a patient with known breast cancer (*E*).

Enhancement kinetics are evaluated in 2 phases, the initial phase and the delayed phase (**Fig. 14**). The initial phase is within the first 2 minutes and is described as slow, medium, or fast. Slow initial phase enhancement is a less than 50% increase in signal intensity. Medium initial phase enhancement is a 50% to 100% increase, and fast initial phase enhancement is a greater than 100% increase in signal intensity. The delayed phase is described as persistent, plateau, or washout. Persistent enhancement is continuously increasing. Plateau enhancement demonstrates no change after the initial phase, and washout shows decreasing signal intensity.

The most suspicious kinetic feature should be reported, because any one lesion may display many different types of kinetic enhancement. Although some studies have shown malignant lesions are more likely to demonstrate washout

kinetics,[12,14,17] others have not found kinetics to be significant predictors of malignancy.[11,16] It is for this reason that the morphology of the lesion should be the most important factor for deciding

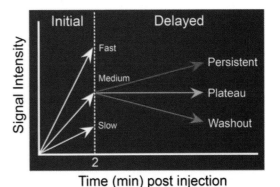

Fig. 14. Kinetic curve assessment.

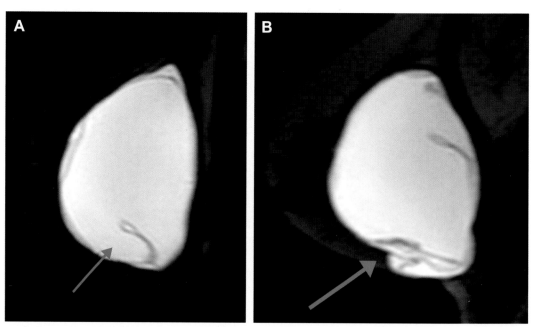

Fig. 15. Signs of intracapsular implant rupture. Sagittal silicone-specific sequences demonstrate the keyhole sign (*A*) and the linguine sign (*B*), annotated by the *red arrows*. Note the white ball at the end of the keyhole sign compared with the black ball seen on the radial fold in **Fig. 16**.

if a lesion requires additional evaluation or biopsy. For example, an intramammary lymph node may display a washout pattern, but the morphology is classic for a common, benign entity that should not be referred for additional evaluation or biopsy.

IMPLANT ASSESSMENT

The section on implant assessment is also new for this edition of BI-RADS. Implant evaluation cannot be adequately performed on a standard breast MR imaging because a dedicated protocol consisting of water and silicone-specific sequences is required, and images in 2 planes should be reviewed, because single plane "ruptures" may simply be a fold in the implant.[18] Evaluation of implants includes a description of lumen type (single lumen vs double lumen), location (prepectoral or retropectoral), and any findings to suggest rupture or signs of implant complications. Intracapsular rupture occurs when the implant ruptures, but the fibrous capsule formed by the body around the implant remains intact. The intact fibrous capsule keeps the silicone from extending into the adjacent breast tissue, and the implant shape may seem to be normal mammographically. MR imaging signs of intracapsular rupture include the subcapsular line, keyhole sign, and the linguine sign (**Fig. 15**). It important to differentiate these signs of intracapsular rupture from the normal undulations of the implant, also known as radial folds (**Fig. 16**). A radial

fold has a dark ball at the end of the fold, whereas the keyhole sign has a white ball at the end owing to the silicone that is outside of the implant settling between the layers of the collapsing implant wall. Extracapsular implant rupture occurs when both the implant wall and the fibrous capsule have broken, and silicone is extruding into the adjacent breast tissue (**Fig. 17**).[18,19] With silicone-sensitive sequences, extracapsular silicone can also be detected in the axillary lymph nodes. Also sometimes seen is a periimplant fluid collection, which can be present in recent implantation,

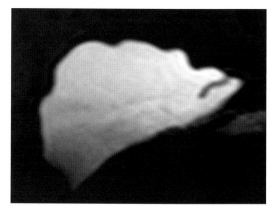

Fig. 16. Radial fold. Axial silicone-specific sequence shows a dark line with a black ball at the end along the medial aspect of the implant.

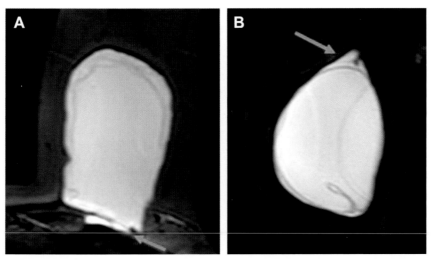

Fig. 17. Signs of extracapsular rupture, annotated by *red arrows*. Axial silicone-specific sequence (*A*) shows extracapsular extrusion of silicone along the chest wall. Also note the subcapsular line along the anterior portion of the implant. Sagittal silicone-specific sequence (*B*) shows extracapsular extrusion of silicone along the superior aspect of the implant.

bleeding, and infection (**Fig. 18**). Although very rare, it is important to be aware of the occurrence of breast implant–associated anaplastic large cell lymphoma. In March 2017, the US Food and Drug Administration released a report detailing 359 medical device reports of breast implant–associated anaplastic large cell lymphoma, including 9 deaths.[20] A recent article by Srinivasa and colleagues[21] reviewed reports from 40 countries and identified 340 unique cases of breast implant–associated anaplastic large cell lymphoma with 5 associated deaths. Both groups

identified a higher incidence in patients with textured surface implants. The most common presentation is a persistent seroma with delayed onset from the time of implantation, although some patients did present with a mass.[20,21]

FINAL ASSESSMENT

Just as with mammography and ultrasound examinations, a final BI-RADS assessment category should be assigned for each study. The final assessment categories are the same for MR

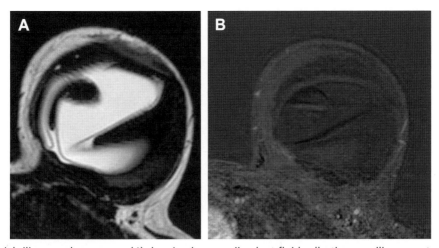

Fig. 18. Axial silicone only sequence (*A*) showing large periimplant fluid collection, no silicone rupture, and the pattern from the textured implants visible along the edges of the implant. Subtraction image (*B*) showing no enhancement within the fluid collection. The fluid was aspirated for preoperative cytology and microbiology studies revealing no evidence of infection or malignancy.

imaging, as for mammography and ultrasound examination:

Category 0: Incomplete, need additional imaging evaluation
Category 1: Negative
Category 2: Benign
Category 3: Probably benign
Category 4: Suspicious
Category 5: Highly suspicious of malignancy
Category 6: Known biopsy-proven malignancy

Although not currently mandated by the US Food and Drug Administration, assigning a final BI-RADS code to each examination is encouraged to aid in communication and provide continuity between mammogram, ultrasound, and MR imaging reports. Of note, implant assessment MR imaging studies should not have a final BI-RADS assessment.

SUMMARY

The updated breast MR imaging BI-RADS lexicon serves to unite terminology and recommendations across multiple modalities, improving communication between radiologists and referring providers. The unification of terminology eliminated confusing or underused descriptors in favor of terms recognized from other, more established modality lexicons. Consistency in reporting improves patient care by providing guidelines for lesion management.

REFERENCES

1. American College of Radiology. Breast Imaging Reporting and Data System (BI-RADS). 1st edition. Reston (VA): American College of Radiology; 1992.
2. American College of Radiology. Breast Imaging Reporting and Data System (BI-RADS). 4th edition. Reston (VA): American College of Radiology; 2003.
3. Morris EA, Comstock CE, Lee CH, et al. ACR BI-RADS® magnetic resonance imaging. In: ACR BI-RADS® atlas, Breast Imaging Reporting and Data System. Reston (VA): American College of Radiology; 2013.
4. McGuire KP. Breast anatomy and physiology. In: Aydiner A, Igci A, Soran A, editors. Breast disease: diagnosis and pathology. New York: Springer International Publishing; 2016. p. 1–14.
5. Giess CS, Yeh ED, Raza S, et al. Background parenchymal enhancement at breast MR imaging: normal patterns, diagnostic challenges, and potential for false-positive and false-negative interpretation. Radiographics 2014;34:234–47.
6. Hambly NM, Liberman L, Dershaw DD, et al. Background parenchymal enhancement on baseline screening breast MRI: impact on biopsy rate and short-interval follow-up. AJR Am J Roentgenol 2011;196:218–24.
7. DeMartini WB, Liu F, Peacock S, et al. Background parenchymal enhancement on breast MRI: impact on diagnostic performance. AJR Am J Roentgenol 2012;198:W373–80.
8. Ha R, Sung J, Lee C, et al. Characteristics and outcome of enhancing foci followed on breast MRI with management implications. Clin Radiol 2014;69:715–20.
9. Liberman L, Mason G, Morris EA, et al. Does size matter? Positive predictive value of MRI-detected breast lesions as a function of lesion size. AJR Am J Roentgenol 2006;186:426–30.
10. Clauser P, Cassano E, De Nicolo A, et al. Foci on breast magnetic resonance imaging in high-risk women: cancer or not? Radiol Med 2016;121:611–7.
11. Liberman L, Morris E, Lee M, et al. Breast lesions detected on MR imaging: features and positive predictive value. AJR Am J Roentgenol 2002;179:171–8.
12. Baltzer P, Benndorf M, Dietzel M, et al. False-positive findings at contrast-enhanced breast MRI: a BI-RADS descriptor study. AJR Am J Roentgenol 2010;194:1658–63.
13. Nunes L, Schnall M, Orel S. Update of breast MR imaging architectural interpretation model. Radiology 2001;219:484–94.
14. Gity M, Moghadam K, Jalali A, et al. Association of different MRI BIRADS descriptors with malignancy in non mass-like breast lesions. Iran Red Crescent Med J 2014;16(12):e26040.
15. Tozaki M, Fukuda K. High-spatial-resolution MRI of non-masslike breast lesions: interpretation model based on BI-RADS MRI descriptors. AJR Am J Roentgenol 2006;187:330–7.
16. Uematsu T, Kasami M. High-spatial-resolution 3T breast MRI on nonmasslike enhancement lesion: an analysis of their features as significant predictors of malignancy. AJR Am J Roentgenol 2012;198:1223–30.
17. Tozaki M, Igarashi T, Fukuda K. Breast MRI using the VIBE sequence: clustered ring enhancement in the differential diagnosis of the lesions showing nonmasslike enhancement. AJR Am J Roentgenol 2006;187:313–21.
18. Shah M, Tanna N, Margolies L. Magnetic resonance imaging of breast implants. Top Magn Reson Imaging 2014;23:345–53.
19. Gorczyca D, Gorczyca S, Gorczyca K. The diagnosis of silicone breast implant rupture. Plast Reconstr Surg 2007;120(7 Suppl 1):49S–61S.
20. US Food and Drug Administration. Breast implant-associated anaplastic large cell lymphoma (BIA-ALCL). 2017. Available at: www.fda.gov. Accessed March 22, 2017.
21. Srinivasa D, Miranda R, Kaura A, et al. Global adverse event reports of breast implant-associated ALCL: an international review of 40 government authority databases. Plast Reconstr Surg 2017;139:1029–39.

Role of MR Imaging for the Locoregional Staging of Breast Cancer

Kimberly M. Ray, MD[a],*, Jessica H. Hayward, MD[b],
Bonnie N. Joe, MD, PhD[b]

KEYWORDS

• Breast MR imaging • Extent of disease • Lymph nodes • Tomosynthesis

KEY POINTS

- In women with newly diagnosed breast cancer, breast MR imaging identifies unsuspected sites of cancer in the ipsilateral breast in 16% of women.
- Breast MR imaging identifies occult cancer in the contralateral breast in 3% to 5% of women with newly diagnosed breast cancer.
- MR imaging is complementary to ultrasound imaging in evaluating the regional nodal basins of women with breast cancer.
- The added value of MR imaging may be attenuated in women with newly diagnosed breast cancer who also undergo tomosynthesis, particularly those with nondense breasts.
- Ongoing prospective, randomized clinical trials should clarify the impact of preoperative breast MR imaging on clinical outcomes.

INTRODUCTION

Breast MR imaging is an exquisitely sensitive technique that has been shown to be useful for defining disease extent within the affected breast, screening the contralateral breast for occult synchronous cancer, and evaluating the regional nodal basins. However, the routine use of breast MR imaging for the evaluation of patients with newly diagnosed breast cancer remains a highly controversial topic because proof of clinical benefit has not yet been clearly demonstrated. In this article, we summarize the existing data on MR imaging performance in extent of disease evaluation and discuss ongoing clinical trials.

Multifocality and Multicentricity of Breast Cancer

Pathology studies of mastectomy specimens have shown that up to 63% of patients with apparently unifocal breast cancer on mammography and clinical examination harbor additional unsuspected malignant foci in the ipsilateral breast.[1,2] In 43% of cases, unsuspected cancer is located greater than 2 cm from the index lesion.[2] Because of this tendency toward multifocality and multicentricity, lumpectomy alone results in unacceptably high rates of local recurrence and postoperative radiation remains a necessary adjunct to breast-conserving surgery.[3]

The authors have nothing to disclose.
[a] Kaiser Permanente, 3600 Broadway, Oakland, CA 94611, USA; [b] Department of Radiology and Biomedical Imaging, University of California, San Francisco, 1600 Divisadero Street, Room C250, San Francisco, CA 94115, USA
* Corresponding author.
E-mail addresses: kimberly.ray@ucsf.edu; kimberly.ray.md@gmail.com

Magn Reson Imaging Clin N Am 26 (2018) 191–205
https://doi.org/10.1016/j.mric.2017.12.008
1064-9689/18/© 2017 Elsevier Inc. All rights reserved.

Multidisciplinary guidelines from the American College of Surgery, American College of Pathology, and American College of Radiology state that mammographically detected multicentric disease is a contraindication to breast-conserving surgery.[4] Furthermore, tumor-free margins at surgical excision are considered a prerequisite for breast conservation. These guidelines highlight the fact that gross tumor left behind at surgery significantly increases a patient's risk of in-breast recurrence. Imaging plays a key role in defining the extent of disease and reducing the tumor burden to a level that can be controlled with postoperative radiation.

MR IMAGING DETECTION OF ADDITIONAL DISEASE IN THE IPSILATERAL BREAST

Numerous studies have shown the increased sensitivity of MR imaging compared with standard mammographic or ultrasound imaging in determining the true extent of disease in patients newly diagnosed with breast cancer.[4–18] Correlative studies of MR imaging and mastectomy specimens performed by Sardanelli and colleagues[15] proved that MR imaging is capable of depicting the clinically and mammographically occult foci of disease that are detected at histopathology (**Fig. 1**). The overall sensitivity of MR for occult multifocal and multicentric disease was 81% (89% for invasive foci and 40% for in situ disease).

In a metaanalysis of 19 published studies involving 2610 women with breast cancer undergoing preoperative MR imaging, Houssami and colleagues[18] found that MR imaging detected additional disease not suspected at mammography and clinical examination in 16% of women. This result was achieved at a high positive predictive value (PPV) of 66%. Because of its greater sensitivity for additional disease foci in newly diagnosed patients, MR imaging has the potential to help select appropriate candidates for breast conservation and to improve surgical planning, increasing the likelihood of complete disease resection.

It has been suggested that the MR imaging-detected cancer may be less clinically important than mammographically detected disease. However, both modalities detect similar rates of invasive cancer and both detect lesions with a median size of approximately 1.0 cm.[11] Iacconi and colleagues[19] studied the characteristics of 73 multicentric cancers detected only at MR imaging in 2021 consecutive women undergoing preoperative MR imaging. These cancers were most frequently invasive carcinomas smaller than

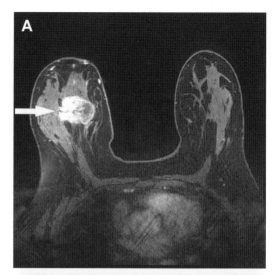

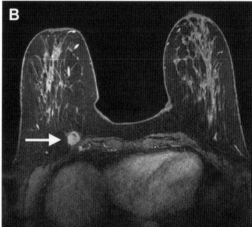

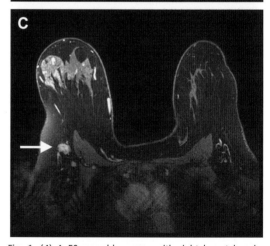

Fig. 1. (*A*) A 50-year-old woman with right breast invasive ductal carcinoma (IDC) presenting as a palpable mass (*arrow*) in the upper central breast shown on MR imaging. (*B*) MR imaging reveals another nonpalpable mass (*arrow*) in the lower central right breast abutting the chest wall, which was not visualized on mammography. Biopsy showed IDC. (*C*) MR imaging also demonstrates right level I axillary adenopathy (*arrow*).

1 cm. However, in 25% of cases the additional cancers were larger than 1 cm, and in 23% of cases the additional disease was larger than the index malignancy. In 3% of cases, the multicentric invasive cancer was of a higher histologic grade than the index invasive cancer. In another 3% of cases, the multicentric invasive cancer was identified in the setting of a known ductal carcinoma in situ (DCIS), altering the disease stage. Hence, the authors concluded that mammographically occult multicentric cancer detected at breast MR imaging seems to represent a greater tumor burden in approximately one-quarter of patients.

CONTRALATERAL DISEASE

The literature also indicates that MR imaging will find mammographically and clinically occult malignancy in the contralateral breast in 3% to 5% of women with a newly diagnosed unilateral breast cancer[20] (**Fig. 2**). In the largest prospective multiinstitutional study published, MR imaging detected 30 contralateral cancers among 969 women with negative mammograms.[21] This added cancer yield was achieved with a PPV of 25%. All of the cancers that were detected by MR imaging were node negative and 40% were DCIS.

Brennan and colleagues[20] performed a systematic review of 22 studies reporting contralateral malignancies detected only by MR imaging in 131 of 3253 women. The incidental contralateral cancer detection rate was 4.1% and the overall PPV was 47.9%. Thirty-five percent of MR imaging-detected cancers were DCIS, 65% were invasive cancers (mean size 9.3 mm), and the majority were node negative.

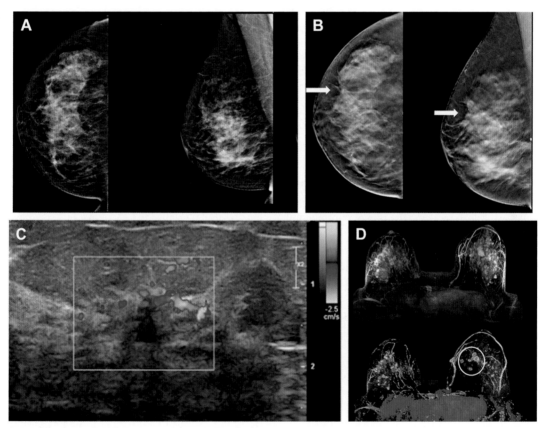

Fig. 2. (*A*) A 41-year-old woman undergoing baseline screening mammography. Standard 2-dimensional craniocaudal (CC; *left*) and mediolateral oblique (MLO; *right*) mammograms were interpreted as negative. (*B*) Architectural distortion (*arrow*) identified in the upper outer right breast on tomosynthesis (CC view [*left*]; MLO view [*right*]). (*C*) Corresponding hypoechoic mass identified on ultrasound imaging (color Doppler image shown). Ultrasound-guided biopsy yielded invasive lobular carcinoma (ILC). (*D*) A 3-dimensional subtracted maximum intensity projection image from contrast-enhanced breast MR imaging demonstrates a marked background parenchymal enhancement. The biopsy-proven cancer in the right breast is significantly masked by the marked background enhancement. However, there are multiple enhancing masses in the inner central left breast (*circled*) with suspicious rapid washout enhancement kinetics (*red*) that represent unsuspected multifocal ILC in the contralateral breast.

Detection of cancer in the opposite breast allows the patient to undergo a single round of treatments for both breasts rather than sequential treatments. This process has obvious psychological, emotional, as well as financial benefits. However, critics of preoperative MR imaging argue that systemic therapies (chemotherapy and endocrine therapy) that are used in the treatment of the ipsilateral cancer may prevent progression of subclinical cancer in the contralateral breast.[22]

Two previous retrospective studies demonstrated no difference in the rate of contralateral breast cancer at 8 to 15 years of follow-up with or without preoperative MR imaging.[23,24] However, these studies were limited to patients undergoing breast-conserving surgery, thereby excluding patients with more advanced disease who might have been at higher risk of contralateral breast cancer. Yi and colleagues[25] retrospectively compared 3440 patients with newly diagnosed breast cancer who underwent preoperative MR imaging, including patients with more advanced cancers, with matched controls without MR imaging. This study showed that preoperative bilateral breast MR imaging was associated with reduced metachronous contralateral breast cancer incidence (0.5% vs 11.0%) at a mean follow-up interval of 65.3 months. Of the 22 metachronous contralateral breast cancers, only 1 node-negative, T1 invasive cancer was detected in the MR imaging group, whereas the remaining 21 cancers detected in the no-MR imaging group varied from stage 0 to 3 and were node positive in 38% of cases. These data suggest that MR imaging can play a role in reducing the rate of contralateral breast cancer.

MR IMAGING COMPARED WITH DIGITAL BREAST TOMOSYNTHESIS FOR LOCAL STAGING

Digital breast tomosynthesis (DBT) is a quasi–3-dimensional mammographic technique that has been shown in multiple clinical studies to have greater sensitivity and specificity than conventional full-field digital mammography (DM).[26] Because DBT is rapidly being incorporated into clinical practice, the incremental benefit of MR imaging in addition to DBT for the local staging of breast cancer warrants evaluation.

Chudgar and colleagues[27] evaluated 82 consecutive patients with screening-detected cancers at DBT who subsequently underwent breast MR imaging for extent of disease evaluation and compared their outcomes with 23 patients with screening-detected cancers at DM who then underwent MR imaging for staging. The proportion of invasive cancers was similar for the DBT and DM groups (73% vs 70%). The DBT group had significantly fewer additional sites of cancer detected at MR imaging (defined as >2 cm from the index lesion or in the contralateral breast; 7/82 [8.5%]) than did the DM group (7/23 [30%]). There were no differences in the proportion of false-positive MR imaging findings between the groups. When the results were stratified by breast density, the additional cancer yield from MR imaging for women with dense breasts was comparable for the DBT and DM groups; however, MR imaging had a significantly reduced benefit for women with nondense breasts in the DBT relative to the DM group.

Mariscotti and colleagues[28] prospectively evaluated 200 consecutive women with breast cancer who underwent screening and diagnostic DM and DBT as well as whole breast ultrasound and MR imaging. They found no difference in sensitivity or accuracy in the preoperative staging of breast cancer whether or not MR imaging was added to the combination of DM + DBT and whole breast ultrasound imaging.

Kim and colleagues[29] conducted a reader study to compare the relative performance of DM alone, DBT plus DM, and MR imaging plus DM in the evaluation of 172 breast cancer cases. The combination of MR imaging plus DM had higher sensitivity than DBT plus DM (97.8% vs 88.2%). However, DBT plus DM showed higher PPV with a lower number of false-positives compared with MR imaging plus DM (93.3% vs 89.6%).

Mercier and colleagues[30] evaluated the performance of DBT relative to DM, ultrasound examination, and MR imaging for breast cancer staging in 75 women with Breast Imaging Reporting and Data System (BIRADS) 4 and 5 lesions. The sensitivities for cancer detection were as follows: 92.5% with MR imaging, 79% for ultrasound examination, 75% for tomosynthesis, and 59.5% for mammography. The treatment plan was altered in 10% of cases owing to additional lesion detection by DBT and in 17% of cases owing to additional detection by MR imaging. When stratified by breast density, MR imaging had significantly greater sensitivity than DBT alone in women with nonfatty breasts (defined as American College of Radiology density categories of scattered, heterogeneously dense, and extremely dense; **Fig. 3**).

Taken together, these early studies suggest that the incremental benefit of MR imaging for local staging of newly diagnosed breast cancer is likely to be attenuated in patients who have undergone DBT. However, the data also suggest that the benefit of MR imaging is likely to remain substantial for women with dense breasts despite DBT.

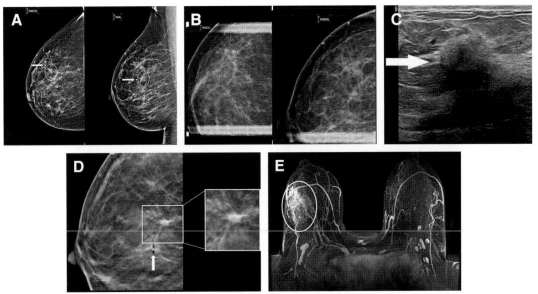

Fig. 3. (*A*) A 51-year-old woman presented with palpable thickening in the outer central right breast, denoted by the metallic BB marker (*arrows*) on 2-dimensional (2D) craniocaudal (CC; *left*) and mediolateral oblique (MLO; *right*) mammograms. A vague focal asymmetry (*circled*) is identified in the area of palpable concern. (*B*) Two-dimensional spot compression magnification mammograms (CC projection shown on left and 90° lateral projection; *right*) over the palpable area show no persistent abnormality. (*C*) Targeted ultrasound imaging of the right breast directed to the palpable area demonstrates a 1.2-cm, indistinct, hypoechoic mass (*arrow*) with posterior shadowing. Subsequent ultrasound-guided biopsy showed fibrocystic change, which was considered a discordant pathology result. (*D*) Subsequent digital breast tomosynthesis shows a 1-cm spiculated mass in the slightly upper outer right breast (*box*) on a 90° lateral projection, which underwent tomosynthesis guided core biopsy yielding invasive lobular carcinoma. A biopsy clip from a prior benign ultrasound-guided biopsy with adjacent artifact is denoted by a white arrow. (*E*) Three-dimensional subtracted maximum intensity projection image from contrast-enhanced bilateral breast MR imaging obtained for extent of disease evaluation demonstrates a 5-cm area of nonmass enhancement (*circled*) in the outer central right breast. MR imaging findings match the extent of disease on final surgical pathology from subsequent lumpectomy.

These findings are expected given the fact that intravenous contrast is not given for DBT and therefore cancers that are embedded in dense breast tissue may remain obscured if there is no margin spiculation or associated architectural distortion.[31,32]

MR IMAGING EVALUATION OF NODAL BASINS

Regional lymph node status is an important component of breast cancer staging, and influences locoregional and systemic treatment decisions.[33,34] Ultrasound imaging is routinely used for the assessment of level I and II axillary lymph nodes, which are most commonly involved in breast cancer. A recent metaanalysis of studies involving 9212 patients with breast cancer demonstrated that the combination of ultrasound examination and ultrasound-guided fine-needle aspiration or core biopsy identified axillary nodal metastases preoperatively in approximately one-half of the patients.[35] However, the false-negative rate was 25%, indicating the necessity of sentinel lymph node biopsy in those cases that are negative on imaging evaluation.

Because of its expanded field of view, MR imaging is complementary to ultrasound examination, permitting evaluation of the level III axillary nodes as well as the extraaxillary basins (**Fig. 4**). In addition, MR imaging is less operator dependent than ultrasound examination. A recent single-institution study (n = 271) showed that MR imaging had superior performance to ultrasound imaging in axillary staging.[36] In this study, MR imaging identified axillary metastases in 15% of patients with initially negative axillary ultrasound examinations. Conversely, only 4% of cases that were negative at MR imaging and deemed positive on ultrasound examination actually proved to be true positive. Overall false-negative rates for MR imaging and axillary ultrasound imaging were 12% and 14%, respectively. Thus, neither modality has a sufficiently high negative predictive value to obviate sentinel node biopsy.

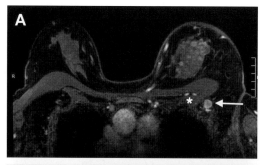

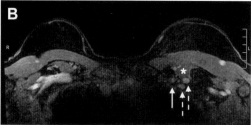

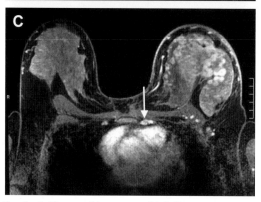

Fig. 4. A 43-year-old woman with inflammatory carcinoma of the left breast with (*A*) level I (*arrow*), (*B*) level II (*dashed white arrows*), and level III (*solid white arrow*) adenopathy. Note that level II nodes are deep to the pectoralis minor muscle (*asterisk*), whereas levels I and III nodes are located lateral and medial, respectively, to the pectoralis minor muscle. (*C*) Internal mammary adenopathy (*arrow*) is also present.

Suspicious lymph node features at MR imaging according to the 5th edition BIRADS lexicon include loss of the fatty hilum, heterogeneous enhancement, and a not circumscribed margin.[37] Several small studies have investigated the predictive value of MR imaging features for nodal metastasis. Baltzer and colleagues[38] correlated MR imaging features of lymph nodes with final pathology in 56 patients with breast cancer and found the best predictors of metastasis to be irregular margin, inhomogeneous cortex, perinodal edema, and asymmetry between the axillae. In a similar study, Mortellaro and colleagues[39] examined 56 patients and found an absence of the fatty hilum to be predictive of metastasis, but not

kinetics, node number, or node size. Because no MR imaging criteria are sufficiently predictive of metastasis, abnormal appearing lymph nodes at MR imaging should undergo sampling under ultrasound guidance before a change in clinical management.

Internal mammary lymph nodes (IMLN) are well seen on breast MR imaging[40] and are important for staging and treatment decisions, because IMLN metastasis is a known poor prognostic factor.[41–43] IMLN metastases are more common in larger primary tumors, especially those located in the medial breast, tumors with lymphovascular invasion, and in younger patients.[27] If IMLN disease is established, additional treatment with targeted radiotherapy and adjuvant chemotherapy may be considered. In the context of a known malignancy, Kinoshita and colleagues[44] found a size threshold of 5 mm had a sensitivity of 93.3% and specificity of 89.3%. However, women without breast cancer undergoing screening MR imaging may have IMLNs with long axis measurements ranging from 2 to 10 mm.[45,46] Because tissue sampling of IMLNs is not routinely performed and treatment of IMLN metastasis may have significant associated morbidity, care should be taken before assessing IMLNs as pathologic on the basis of imaging. Morphology may be helpful to distinguish benign from malignant nodes. In 1 series, all incidental benign nodes had fatty hila and/or oval shape with circumscribed margins.[46] IMLN metastases without concomitant axillary nodal metastases are rare,[47] particularly in lateral tumors. PET/computed tomography may be helpful for confirmation in equivocal cases.[40,48]

IMPACT OF BREAST MR IMAGING ON SURGICAL OUTCOMES

Randomized, controlled trials have demonstrated equivalent disease-free and overall survivals as well as equivalent local recurrence rates for women undergoing lumpectomy with radiation compared with mastectomy.[3,49–51] However, approximately one-quarter of all patients who undergo breast-conserving surgery in the United States, an estimated 20,000 women annually, will require an additional operation to achieve negative margins.[52] This step adds significant financial and psychological burdens for women seeking breast conservation and may also lead to less favorable cosmetic outcomes. Higher repeat surgery rates are more common in patients who are younger, have larger tumors, and/or have a lobular histology.

More accurate local staging of disease through breast MR imaging presents an opportunity to improve surgical outcomes. MR imaging detects additional sites of disease that are occult to mammography and clinical examination in approximately 16% of women with newly diagnosed breast cancer. As a direct consequence of this increased detection, preoperative breast MR imaging alters surgical management in 8% to 20% of patients.[18] In 1 metaanalysis, the rate of conversion from wide local excision to mastectomy was 8.1% and to more extensive surgery was 11.3%.[18] Changes in surgical management were not always appropriate: 1% of women were converted to mastectomy and 5.5% converted from wide local excision to more extensive excision or mastectomy based on false-positive MR imaging findings. Such data reinforce the importance of basing surgical management decisions on biopsy-proven lesions and not merely a suspicious appearance on MR imaging.

In a subsequent metaanalysis of 9 studies (2 randomized trials and 7 comparative cohorts) that compared preoperative MR imaging with conventional imaging with a total of 3112 subjects, there was a 7.3% increase in the overall mastectomy rate in the MR imaging group. This increase was due to a higher rate of mastectomy as the initial surgery in the MR imaging group rather than as a follow-up to lumpectomy with positive margins.[53] Surprisingly, despite the increase in initial mastectomies, MR imaging did not significantly decrease the proportion of patients with incomplete excision or the odds of reoperation.

The apparent lack of benefit from MR imaging in the described metaanalysis[53] might be explained by a number of compromising factors. The majority of studies included were retrospective and, therefore, were inherently subject to selection bias. For example, in all 7 of the retrospective studies,[54–60] the women who underwent MR imaging were younger than those who did not undergo MR imaging. Furthermore, MR imaging–guided core biopsy was not always available to establish the histopathology of MR imaging findings. Finally, the manner in which surgeons incorporated suspicious preoperative MR imaging findings into their surgical approach was highly variable.

Two prospective, randomized, controlled trials comparing the effect of preoperative MR imaging with conventional imaging on surgical outcomes have been performed[61,62] and were included in the described metaanalysis. The COMICE (Comparative Effectiveness of MR imaging in Breast Cancer) trial[61] was conducted in the UK from 2002 to 2007, enrolling 1623 women from 45 centers. The trial found that there was no in the reoperation rate with or without the use of MR imaging. There were several significant limitations of the COMICE trial. Although the trial was prospective in design, there was very low recruitment from a number of participating centers, which introduces potential selection bias. Low-volume centers may also have lacked expertise in the performance and interpretation of breast MR imaging. MR imaging–guided tissue sampling was unavailable at some centers, one consequence of which was a number of inappropriate mastectomies for false-positive findings. Finally, a major limitation of COMICE was the lack of a systematic approach to incorporating MR imaging findings into the surgical plan, which would have diminished the potential impact of MR imaging.

The MONET (MR mammography of nonpalpable breast tumors) trial[62] was a randomized controlled trial in which patients with nonpalpable BIRADS 3, 4, or 5 lesions were randomly assigned to undergo mammography, ultrasound imaging, and biopsy versus additional MR imaging before biopsy. Four hundred eighteen patients were randomized. Among the 149 patients with biopsy-proven malignancies, there was a paradoxically higher reexcision rate in the MR imaging group. Because the MONET trial only included patients with nonpalpable lesions, 60% of cases were mammographically detected calcifications and one-half of the cancers were DCIS in both the study and control groups. In contrast, DCIS would only account for one-quarter of breast malignancies in the general population. Therefore, the findings from the MONET trial are not generalizable to all women with breast cancer. Furthermore, as in the COMICE trial, the findings at preoperative MR imaging were not applied to the surgical plan in a systematic manner, thus limiting the potential benefit from MR imaging.

In a more recent retrospective study, Sung and colleagues[40] compared 174 consecutive women who underwent preoperative MR imaging with a control group that did not undergo MR imaging, and were matched by age at diagnosis, tumor stage, histopathologic features, and surgeon. MR imaging findings were incorporated into the surgical decision making for all women in the MR imaging group. The study demonstrated that significantly fewer women in the MR imaging group needed reexcision than those without MR imaging (29% vs 45%). Although limited to outcomes from a single institution, this study provides evidence that the deliberate application of MR imaging findings to surgical planning can have a substantial impact on surgical outcomes.

One of the objectives of the ongoing Alliance A011104/American College of Radiology Imaging Network (ACRIN) 6694 multicenter, prospective, randomized controlled trial of preoperative MR imaging[63] is to establish standards for the interpretation, reporting, and clinical implementation of MR imaging findings. Such programmatic guidelines are key to ensuring the effective translation of information from MR imaging to the operating room. Forthcoming results of this trial should more definitively address the effect of preoperative MR imaging on surgical outcomes.

IMPACT OF MR IMAGING ON MASTECTOMY RATES

Preoperative breast MR imaging has been criticized for leading to overtreatment and especially for increasing the rate of mastectomies.[53,64,65] To a certain extent, conversion to mastectomy for a subset of patients on the basis of MR imaging findings is expected and appropriate given that in approximately 10% of patients MR imaging detects mammographically occult multicentric disease, which is a contraindication to breast conservation.

However, a number of retrospective studies that have reported an association between the use of preoperative MR imaging and increased mastectomy rates have been significantly limited owing to their failure to control for a number of variables that may be independently associated with mastectomy rates.[66–68] It has been shown that women who tend to undergo preoperative MR imaging are more likely to be young, have dense breasts, and to be at higher risk owing to genetic mutations or other factors.[69–71] They also tend to have more aggressive tumor subtypes and are more likely to be treated at academic centers that offer breast reconstruction. Many of these variables are also likely to influence decisions regarding mastectomy.[72]

A study from the Mayo Clinic of more than 5000 patients with breast cancer who underwent surgery between 1997 and 2006 suggests there are factors besides MR imaging contributing to increasing mastectomy rates.[67] Mastectomy rates decreased from 1997 to 2003, but subsequently increased from 2004 to 2006. The increase in mastectomies coincided with a doubling in the rate of preoperative MR imaging. However, although patients with MR imaging were more likely to undergo mastectomy than those without MR imaging (54% vs 36%), further analysis revealed that mastectomy rates increased in all patients from 2004 to 2006, and did so predominantly among patients who did not undergo MR imaging.

Tuttle and colleagues[73] reported data from the Surveillance, Epidemiology, and End Results database showing that the use of contralateral prophylactic mastectomy among patients with unilateral invasive breast cancer more than doubled from 1998 to 2003. This period preceded the widespread clinical use of MR imaging, and thus points to the importance of other factors driving the trend toward increased mastectomies. For example, the authors noted a concurrent increase in reconstructive procedures during the study period. Similarly, the ACRIN 6667 multicenter preoperative breast MR imaging trial found that false-positive MR imaging results did not increase the rates of contralateral prophylactic mastectomy.[71] In contrast, younger age, family history, breast density, and having DCIS as the index cancer were all positively associated with an increased contralateral mastectomy rate.

In summary, decision making regarding mastectomy depends on a complex interplay of factors, including but not limited to the use of breast MR imaging. Further studies are needed to clarify the precise impact of these different variables on patient and clinician decision making.

INVASIVE LOBULAR CARCINOMA

Invasive lobular cancer (ILC) accounts for approximately 10% to 14% of invasive breast carcinomas.[74] The mammogram is more often falsely negative in invasive lobular than in invasive ductal cancer because of the tendency of the cells to grow in a single file arrangement in ILC.[75] ILC also has a higher frequency of multicentricity and bilaterality than invasive ductal cancer.[76] Because of the difficulty in determining the extent of ILC, reported reexcision rates are high, ranging from 29% to 67%.[77–81]

MR imaging has shown greater accuracy in depicting the extent of ILC compared with mammography. In a metaanalysis of 6 studies totaling 220 patients, the estimated correlation coefficient relating MR imaging size estimation of ILC to pathologic size was 0.89 as compared with 0.27 for mammography.[82] This was due in part to the greater sensitivity of MR imaging for multifocal and multicentric disease, which was present in approximately one-third of patients.[83–85]

In another metaanalysis[53] that included 766 patients with ILC, there was a trend toward reduced reexcision rates after initial breast conservation in patients that underwent preoperative MR imaging (10.9% vs 18.0%), although this did not attain statistical significance. The overall mastectomy rate was significantly higher in the MR imaging group (43.0% vs 40.2%).

In a retrospective cohort study of 267 consecutive ILC patients presenting at 2 tertiary cancer centers, Mann and colleagues[58,86] reported that the reexcision rate in 99 patients who underwent preoperative MR imaging was significantly lower than in the no-MR imaging group (9% vs 27%). In addition, there was a trend toward a lower final mastectomy rate in the MR imaging versus no-MR imaging group (48 vs 59%). These results suggest that, at centers with expertise, MR imaging does have the potential to improve surgical outcomes for patients with ILC.

Ductal Carcinoma In Situ and Extensive Intraductal Component

DCIS accounts for approximately one-quarter of all breast malignancies that are diagnosed in the United States.[71] Although DCIS itself lacks metastatic potential, approximately one-half of the recurrences that arise after resection of DCIS are invasive carcinomas.[87] Thus, it is imperative to achieve adequate local control of DCIS. The presence of positive margins after breast-conserving surgery for DCIS is one of the strongest predictors of local recurrence.[87–89] Furthermore, in 30% to 40% of all invasive breast carcinomas, there is an extensive intraductal component (EIC), defined as when DCIS involves more than 25% of the invasive tumor and extends into the surrounding tissue. EIC is associated with an increased recurrence rate, which is likely due to residual disease.[90]

Mammography has been shown to underestimate the extent of DCIS. In a retrospective study of 2564 patients with DCIS, Thomas and colleagues[91] found that mammography underestimated disease extent in 30% of patients undergoing breast-conserving surgery. Dillon and colleagues[92] showed that there was a discrepancy of more than 1 cm between mammography and pathology in 40% of patients who had positive surgical margins compared with only 14% of patients with negative margins.

Over the past decade, a shift in emphasis toward higher spatial resolution protocols has enabled MR imaging to surpass mammography in sensitivity for the detection of DCIS[92–94] and accuracy in estimation of pathologic size.[95,96] In a large, prospective, observational study (n = 7319) of patients that underwent both mammography and MR imaging evaluation of pure DCIS, Kuhl and colleagues[97] found that 48% of DCIS was missed by mammography, but detected on MR imaging. In patients with high-grade or comedo-type DCIS, the sensitivity of MR imaging was 98% compared with only 52% for mammography. Conversely, the majority (83%) of DCIS cases that were falsely negative on MR imaging were non–high-grade lesions.

MR imaging has been shown to change the surgical management of DCIS. Berg and colleagues[93] reported on a series of 38 DCIS lesions, of which 34 (89%) were detected by MR imaging, as compared with 21 (55%) at mammography. Two of the 12 cases (17%) were appropriately converted from breast-conserving surgery to mastectomy on the basis of MR imaging findings. Of the 19 cases with EIC, the EIC was only depicted at MR imaging in 6 cases (32%). Because breast conservation was planned for 5 of the 6 cases with MR imaging-depicted EIC, the additional information provided by MR imaging would have been expected to affect surgical planning for these patients.

Hollingsworth and colleagues[98] investigated the frequency of occult invasion in 288 consecutive patients with newly diagnosed DCIS. At preoperative MR imaging, unsuspected foci of invasive cancer, either multicentric or contralateral, were identified in 3.5% of cases. The discovery of invasive disease at MR imaging alters disease staging and enables sentinel node biopsy to be performed at the time of lumpectomy.

Although MR imaging provides more accurate mapping of disease extent, evidence regarding the impact of MR imaging on positive margins is mixed. In a retrospective cohort study by Allen and colleagues[99] (n = 98), there were fewer cases of positive margins among patients who underwent preoperative MR imaging compared with those who did not undergo MR imaging (21.2% vs 30.8%), although this finding did not attain statistical significance. However, Kropcho and colleagues[100] (n = 158) found that, although tumor size assessment by MR imaging was strongly correlated with histopathologic size, preoperative MR imaging did not reduce the rate of positive margins. In the latter study, the lack of surgical benefit despite the greater accuracy of MR imaging points to the difficulty in applying MR imaging findings in the operating room.

False-positive findings in the preoperative MR imaging evaluation of DCIS are common. Overestimation of size of DCIS or EIC at MR imaging has been reported in up to 50% of cases.[91,95,101,102] Kumar and colleagues[103] reported that MR imaging overestimated disease extent by 200% or more in mostly non–high-grade and non–comedo-type DCIS. Because of the risk of false-positive findings on MR imaging, tissue sampling should be considered mandatory before recommending a change in surgical management.

In the MONET randomized controlled trial,[62] 418 patients were assigned to undergo either mammography and ultrasound examination or MR imaging before biopsy. Because only nonpalpable findings were included, there was a high proportion (60%) of calcification-only findings in the study cohort. A paradoxically higher rate of reexcision owing to positive margins after initial breast-conserving surgery was seen in patients who underwent preoperative MR imaging relative to the control group (34% vs 12%). The reoperation rate was highest in women who had negative MR imaging findings (11/17), and the majority of these patients had DCIS (10/11). This observation suggests MR imaging was falsely reassuring in cases of calcified DCIS without an MR imaging correlate, and may have led to performance of smaller excisions, resulting in an increased rate of positive margins. In fact, the median excision volume of DCIS cases without MR imaging correlate was one-half the size of cases with a correlate.

Taken together, these studies indicate that MR imaging is complementary to mammography for mapping the extent of DCIS. Further studies are needed to determine which subsets of women with DCIS will gain the most benefit from MR imaging. As is true for preoperative MR imaging in general, clinical outcomes for women with DCIS who undergo MR imaging evaluation are greatly dependent on the manner in which MR imaging findings are applied in the surgical setting. The wide variation in clinical outcomes in studies to date highlights the need for guidelines regarding the application of MR imaging findings at surgery.

IMPACT OF MR IMAGING ON RECURRENCE RATES

There are currently no data from prospective, randomized, controlled trials regarding the impact of preoperative breast MR imaging on local recurrence rates. Several nonrandomized, single-institution, retrospective cohort studies have yielded conflicting results. Fischer and colleagues[104] reported on 225 patients who underwent breast conservation. At a mean follow-up interval of 40 months, patients who underwent preoperative MR imaging had a lower rate of local recurrence than patients who did not undergo MR imaging (1.2% vs 6.5%). However, no adjustments for tumor size or nodal status were made between the study groups. Most important, the rate of chemotherapy administration was lower in the non-MR imaging group, which may have accounted for the higher recurrence rate, thus confounding the study results.

Solin and colleagues reported on 755 women treated with breast-conserving surgery, of whom 215 underwent MR imaging.[23,105] Of note, one-half of these 215 patients underwent MR imaging after surgery, which likely had a negative impact on MR imaging performance owing to postoperative changes. There was no difference in the local recurrence rates in the group with or without MR imaging on follow-up at 8 years (3% vs 4%) or 15 years (8% in both groups). In contrast to the study by Fischer and colleagues,[104] the rates of systemic therapies were similar between the study groups. However, given the retrospective design, selection bias cannot be excluded. The women who underwent MR imaging were younger than those in the control group. Not reported were other factors that might have influenced the decision to perform MR imaging, such as high-risk status, dense breast tissue, or equivocal mammograms.

In another retrospective study, Sung and colleagues[24] reported the effect of preoperative MR imaging on the outcomes of 174 women with early stage breast cancer. Women in the study group who underwent MR imaging and those in the control group were matched by age, histopathologic findings, surgeon, and stage. The rates of adjuvant systemic and radiation therapy were also similar between the 2 groups. With a median follow-up of 8 years, there was no difference in locoregional recurrence rate between the MR imaging and no-MR imaging groups (5% vs 9%). The authors of this study noted that selection bias could have affected their results. In particular, women in the preoperative MR imaging group were more likely to have dense breasts and bilateral breast cancer.

Gervais and colleagues[106] published a retrospective study of 470 patients, of which 27% underwent preoperative breast MR imaging and 73% did not. The MR imaging group was younger, more frequently received adjuvant chemotherapy, presented with larger tumors, and had a greater proportion of human epidermal growth factor receptor 2 (HER2)–positive and triple-negative (estrogen and progesterone receptor-negative, HER2-negative) cancers. There was no difference in the local recurrence rate at 10 years between those who received MR imaging versus those who did not (1.6% vs 4.2%), even after adjusting for age, year of surgery, tumor size, and adjuvant treatments.

In summary, because of the lack of prospective, randomized, controlled trials, the potential of MR imaging to affect local recurrence rates is uncertain. All previous retrospective studies have been subject to selection bias, whereby the women selected to undergo MR imaging may have been at higher risk of recurrence to begin with. The data indicate that the overall recurrence rates in a general population of women with early stage breast cancer are low (<10%), and therefore MR imaging is not likely to offer significant benefit for all women. However, future prospective trials are needed to determine whether certain subgroups of women, including those who are younger, have a higher risk status, or more aggressive tumors may gain significant benefit from preoperative MR imaging.

IMPACT OF MR IMAGING IN THE CONTEXT OF MOLECULAR SUBTYPES

Molecular profiling studies have revealed breast cancer to be a heterogeneous disease, which is composed of 4 distinct subtypes that have different clinical behaviors and responses to treatment. There is emerging evidence that breast cancer subtypes may predict locoregional recurrence. Specifically, HER2-enriched and basal subtypes have been shown to be associated with an increased risk of locoregional recurrence relative to the luminal A subtype.[107,108] It is currently unknown whether increased recurrence rates for these tumor subtypes reflect inadequate local treatment or are the consequence of biologically aggressive disease.

MR imaging has been shown to identify unexpected foci of disease in patients with aggressive tumor subtypes and may have a role in improving local control. In a study of 299 women undergoing preoperative MR imaging, Ha and colleagues[109] found the Erb-B2 receptor tyrosine kinase 2 (also known as HER2-enriched) and luminal B subtypes were more often associated with multifocal and multicentric disease, skin and nipple–areolar involvement, and axillary nodal disease than were luminal A cancers. Gervais and colleagues[106] found that, among patients who underwent preoperative MR imaging, there was no difference in the 10-year local recurrence rate between women with high-risk cancers (defined as triple negative and HER2 positive) and other subtypes. Interestingly, however, within the group that did not undergo MR imaging, the recurrence rate was higher in the high-risk tumor group, although this difference did not attain statistical significance. The authors concluded that there may be an association between performing preoperative MR imaging and reducing the local recurrence rate in the high-risk tumor subgroup, because MR imaging may identify additional lesions that could be clinically relevant in this specific population.

The ongoing Alliance A011104/ACRIN 6694 randomized controlled trial[63] comparing mammography (with or without ultrasound examination) alone versus in combination with preoperative MR imaging for local staging specifically targets women with triple-negative and HER2-positive tumors. The investigators hypothesize that these patients are at the highest risk of local recurrence owing to increased rates of multifocality and multicentricity. The potential of preoperative MR imaging to reduce local recurrence owing to more effective disease mapping is most likely to be maximized in this patient cohort.

SUMMARY

Breast MR imaging is a highly sensitive technique that has the potential to improve the local staging of breast cancer if systematically applied in properly selected patients. Hopefully, ongoing prospective randomized clinical trials will clarify the effects of preoperative MR imaging on surgical outcomes, costs, and quality of life.

REFERENCES

1. Holland R, Hendriks JH, Mravunac M. Mammographically occult breast cancer. A pathologic and radiologic study. Cancer 1983;52(10):1810–9.
2. Holland R, Veling SMJ, Mravunac M, et al. Histologic multifocality of Tis, T1, T1-2 breast carcinomas: implication for clinical trials of breast-conserving surgery. Cancer 1985;56:979–90.
3. Early Breast Cancer Trialists' Collaborative Group. Effects of radiotherapy and surgery in early breast cancer. An overview of the randomized trials. N Engl J Med 1995;333:1444–55.
4. Harms SE, Flamig DP. MR imaging of the breast: technical approach and clinical experience. Radiographics 1993;13:905–12.
5. Orel SG, Schnall MD, Powell CM, et al. Staging of suspected breast cancer: effect of MR imaging and MR-guided biopsy. Radiology 1995;196:115–22.
6. Mumtaz H, Hall-Craggs MA, Davidson T, et al. Staging of symptomatic primary breast cancer with MR imaging. AJR Am J Roentgenol 1997;169:417–24.
7. Fischer U, Kopka L, Grabbe E. Breast carcinoma: effect of preoperative contrast-enhanced MR imaging on the therapeutic approach. Radiology 1999;213:881–8.
8. Bedrosian I, Mick R, Orel SG, et al. Changes in the surgical management of patients with breast carcinoma based on preoperative magnetic resonance imaging. Cancer 2003;98:468–73.
9. Liberman L, Morris EA, Dershaw DD, et al. MR imaging of the ipsilateral breast in women with percutaneously proven breast cancer. AJR Am J Roentgenol 2003;180:901–9.
10. Schelfout K, Van Goethem M, Kersschot E, et al. Contrast-enhanced MR imaging of breast lesions and effect on treatment. Eur J Surg Oncol 2004;30:501–7.

11. Schnall MD, Blume J, Bluemke DA, et al. MRI detection of distinct incidental cancer in women with primary breast cancer studied in IBMC 6883. J Surg Oncol 2005;92:32–8.

12. Tan JE, Orel SG, Schnall MD, et al. Role of magnetic resonance imaging and magnetic resonance imaging— guided surgery in the evaluation of patients with early-stage breast cancer for breast conservation treatment. Am J Clin Oncol 1999;22: 414–8.

13. Tillman GF, Orel SG, Schnall MD, et al. Effect of breast magnetic resonance imaging on the clinical management of women with early-stage breast carcinoma. J Clin Oncol 2002;20:3413–23.

14. Hollingsworth AB, Stough RG, O'Dell CA, et al. Breast magnetic resonance imaging for preoperative locoregional staging. Am J Surg 2008;196: 389–97.

15. Sardanelli F, Giuseppetti GM, Panizza P, et al. Sensitivity of MRI versus mammography for detecting foci of multifocal, multicentric breast cancer in fatty and dense breasts using the whole-breast pathologic examination as a gold standard. AJR Am J Roentgenol 2004;183:1149–57.

16. Hlawatsch A, Teifke A, Schmidt M, et al. Preoperative assessment of breast cancer: sonography versus MR imaging. AJR Am J Roentgenol 2002; 179:1493–501.

17. Bagley FH. The role of magnetic resonance imaging mammography in the surgical management of the index breast cancer. Arch Surg 2004;139: 380–3.

18. Houssami N, Ciatto S, Macaskill P, et al. Accuracy and surgical impact of magnetic resonance imaging in breast cancer staging: systematic review and meta-analysis in detection of multifocal and multicentric cancer. J Clin Oncol 2008;26:3248–58.

19. Iacconi C, Galman L, Zheng J, et al. Multicentric cancer detected at breast MR imaging and not at mammography: important or not? Radiology 2016;279:378–84.

20. Brennan ME, Houssami N, Lord S, et al. Magnetic resonance imaging screening of the contralateral breast in women with newly diagnosed breast cancer: systematic review and meta-analysis of incremental cancer detection and impact on surgical management. J Clin Oncol 2009;27(33):5640–9.

21. Lehman CD, Gatsonis C, Kuhl CK, et al, ACRIN Trial 6667 Investigators Group. MRI evaluation of the contralateral breast in women with recently diagnosed breast cancer. N Engl J Med 2007; 356:1295–303.

22. Early Breast Cancer Trialists' Collaborative Group. Effects of chemotherapy and hormonal therapy for early breast cancer on recurrence and 15-year survival: an overview of the randomised trials. Lancet 2005;365:1687–717.

23. Solin LJ, Orel SG, Hwang WT, et al. Relationship of breast magnetic resonance imaging to outcome after breast-conservation treatment with radiation for women with early-stage invasive breast carcinoma or ductal carcinoma in situ. J Clin Oncol 2008;26: 386–91.

24. Sung JS, Li J, Da Costa G, et al. Preoperative breast MRI for early- stage breast cancer: effect on surgical and long-term outcomes. AJR Am J Roentgenol 2014;202:1376–82.

25. Yi A, Cho N, Yang KS, et al. Breast cancer recurrence in patients with newly diagnosed breast cancer without and with preoperative MR imaging: a matched cohort study. Radiology 2015;276(3): 695–705.

26. Vedantham S, Karellas A, Vijayaraghavan GR, et al. Digital breast tomosynthesis: state of the art. Radiology 2015;277:663–84.

27. Chudgar AV, Conant EF, Weinstein SP, et al. Assessment of disease extent on contrast-enhanced MRI in breast cancer detected at digital breast tomosynthesis versus digital mammography alone. Clin Radiol 2017;72(7):573–9.

28. Mariscotti G, Houssami N, Durando M, et al. Accuracy of mammography, digital breast tomosynthesis, ultrasound and MR imaging in preoperative assessment of breast cancer. Anticancer Res 2014;34:1219–25.

29. Kim WH, Chang JM, Moon H, et al. Comparison of the diagnostic performance of digital breast tomosynthesis and magnetic resonance imaging added to digital mammography in women with known breast cancers. Eur Radiol 2016;26: 1556–64.

30. Mercier J, Kwiatkowski F, Abrial C, et al. The role of tomosynthesis in breast cancer staging in 75 patients. Diagn Interv Imaging 2015;96:27–35.

31. Rafferty EA, Durand MA, Conant EF, et al. Breast cancer screening using tomosynthesis and digital mammography in dense and nondense breasts. JAMA 2016;315(16):1784–6.

32. Conant EF. Clinical implementation of digital breast tomosynthesis. Radiol Clin North Am 2014;52:499–518.

33. Yoshihara E, Smeets A, Laenen A, et al. Predictors of axillary lymph node metastases in early breast cancer and their applicability in clinical practice. Breast 2013;22(3):357–61.

34. Anderson TL, Glazebrook KN, Murphy BL, et al. Cross-sectional imaging to evaluate the extent of regional nodal disease in breast cancer patients undergoing neoadjuvant systemic therapy. Eur J Radiol 2017;89:163–8.

35. Diepstraten SC, Sever AR, Buckens CF, et al. Value of preoperative ultrasound-guided axillary lymph node biopsy for preventing completion axillary lymph node dissection in breast cancer: a

systematic review and meta-analysis. Ann Surg Oncol 2014;21(1):51–9.

36. Assing MA, Patel BK, Karamsadkar N, et al. A comparison of the diagnostic accuracy of magnetic resonance imaging to axillary ultrasound in the detection of axillary nodal metastases in newly diagnosed breast cancer. Breast J 2017;23(6): 647–55.

37. Morris EA, Comstock CE, Lee CH, et al. ACR BI-RADS® magnetic resonance imaging. In: ACR BI-RADS® atlas, breast imaging reporting and data system. Reston (VA): American College of Radiology; 2013.

38. Baltzer PA, Dietzel M, Burmeister HP, et al. Application of MR mammography beyond local staging: is there a potential to accurately assess axillary lymph nodes? Evaluation of an extended protocol in an initial prospective study. AJR 2011;196(5): W641–7.

39. Mortellaro VE, Marshall J, Singer L, et al. Magnetic resonance imaging for axillary staging in patients with breast cancer. J Magn Reson Imaging 2009; 30(2):309–12.

40. Jochelson MS, Lebron L, Jacobs SS, et al. Detection of internal mammary adenopathy in patients with breast cancer by PET/CT and MRI. AJR Am J Roentgenol 2015;205(4):899–904.

41. Chen RC, Lin NU, Golshan M, et al. Internal mammary nodes in breast cancer: diagnosis and implications for patient management – a systematic review. J Clin Oncol 2008;26(30):4981–9.

42. Cody HS 3rd, Urban JA. Internal mammary node status: a major prognosticator in axillary node-negative breast cancer. Ann Surg Oncol 1995;2: 32–7.

43. Veronesi U, Cascinelli N, Greco M, et al. Prognosis of breast cancer patients after mastectomy and dissection of internal mammary nodes. Ann Surg 1985;202:702–7.

44. Kinoshita T, Odagiri K, Andoh K, et al. Evaluation of small internal mammary lymph node metastases in breast cancer by MRI. Radiat Med 1999;17(3): 189–93.

45. Ray KM, Munir R, Wisner DJ, et al. Internal mammary lymph nodes as incidental findings at screening breast MRI. Clin Imaging 2015;39(5): 791–3.

46. Mack M, Chetlen A, Liao J. Incidental internal mammary lymph nodes visualized on screening breast MRI. AJR Am J Roentgenol 2015;205:209–14.

47. Byrd DR, Dunnwald LK, Mankoff DA, et al. Internal mammary lymph node drainage patterns in patients with breast cancer documented by breast lymphoscintigraphy. Ann Surg Oncol 2001;8:234–40.

48. Wang CL, Eissa MJ, Rogers JV, et al. 18F-FDG PET/CT–positive internal mammary lymph nodes: pathologic correlation by ultrasound-guided fine-needle aspiration and assessment of associated risk factors. AJR 2013;200:1138–44.

49. Fisher B, Bauer M, Margolese R, et al. Five-year results of a randomized clinical trial comparing total mastectomy and segmental mastectomy with or without radiation in the treatment of breast cancer. N Engl J Med 1985;312(11):665–73.

50. Fisher B, Anderson S, Bryant J, et al. Twenty-year follow-up of a randomized trial comparing total mastectomy, lumpectomy, and lumpectomy plus irradiation for the treatment of invasive breast cancer. N Engl J Med 2002;347(16):1233–41.

51. van Dongen JA, Voogd AC, Fentiman IS, et al. Long-term results of a randomized trial comparing breast-conserving therapy with mastectomy: European Organization for Research and Treatment of Cancer 10801 trial. J Natl Cancer Inst 2000; 92(14):1143–50.

52. Wilke LG, Czechura T, Wang C, et al. Repeat surgery after breast conservation for the treatment of stage 0 to II breast carcinoma: a report from the National Cancer Data Base, 2004–2010. JAMA Surg 2014;149:1296–305.

53. Houssami N, Turner R, Morrow M. Preoperative magnetic resonance imaging in breast cancer: meta-analysis of surgical outcomes. Ann Surg 2013;257(2):249–55.

54. Pengel KE, Loo CE, Teertstra HJ, et al. The impact of preoperative MRI on breast-conserving surgery of invasive cancer: a comparative cohort study. Breast Cancer Res Treat 2009;116:161–9.

55. Bleicher RJ, Ciocca RM, Egleston BL, et al. Association of routine pretreatment magnetic resonance imaging with time to surgery, mastectomy rate, and margin status. J Am Coll Surg 2009; 294(209):180–7.

56. Hwang N, Schiller DE, Crystal P, et al. Magnetic resonance imaging in the planning of initial lumpectomy for invasive breast carcinoma: its effect on ipsilateral breast tumor recurrence after breast-conservation therapy. Ann Surg Oncol 2009;16:3000–9.

57. Miller B, Abbott A, Tuttle T. The influence of preoperative MRI on breast cancer treatment. Ann Surg Oncol 2012;19:536–40.

58. Mann RM, Loo CE, Wobbes T, et al. The impact of preoperative breast MRI on the re-excision rate in invasive lobular carcinoma of the breast. Breast Cancer Res Treat 2010;119(2):415–22.

59. McGhan LJ, Wasif N, Gray RJ, et al. Use of preoperative magnetic resonance imaging for invasive lobular cancer: good, better, but maybe not the best? Ann Surg Oncol 2010;17(suppl 3):255–62.

60. Heil J, Buhler A, Golatta M, et al. Does a supplementary preoperative breast MRI in patients with invasive lobular breast cancer change primary

and secondary surgical interventions? Ann Surg Oncol 2011;18:2143–9.

61. Turnbull L, Brown S, Harvey I, et al. Comparative effectiveness of MRI in breast cancer (COMICE) trial: a randomised controlled trial. Lancet 2010; 375:563–71.

62. Peters NH, van ES, van den Bosch MA, et al. Pre-operative MRI and surgical management in patients with nonpalpable breast cancer: the MONET— randomised controlled trial. Eur J Cancer 2011;47:879–86.

63. Bedrosian I. Effect of preoperative breast MRI on surgical outcomes, costs and quality of life of women with breast cancer. ALLIANCE A 0111 04/ACRIN 6694 trial. NC T01805076.

64. Morrow M, Freedman G. A clinical oncology perspective on the use of breast MR. Magn Reson Imaging Clin N Am 2006;14:363–78.

65. Morrow M. Magnetic resonance imaging in the breast cancer patient: curb your enthusiasm. J Clin Oncol 2008;26(3):352–3.

66. Kummerow KL, Du L, Penson DF, et al. Nationwide trends in mastectomy for early-stage breast cancer. JAMA Surg 2015;150(1):9–16.

67. Katipamula R, Degnim AC, Hoskin T, et al. Trends in mastectomy rates at the Mayo Clinic Rochester: effect of surgical year and preoperative magnetic resonance imaging. J Clin Oncol 2009;27(25): 4082–8.

68. Dragun AE, Pan J, Riley EC, et al. Increasing use of elective mastectomy and contralateral prophylactic surgery among breast conservation candidates: a 14-year report from a comprehensive cancer center. Am J Clin Oncol 2013;36(4):375–80.

69. Miller JW, Sabatino S, Thompson TD, et al. Breast MRI use uncommon among U.S. Women. Cancer Epidemiol Biomarkers Prev 2013;22(1):159–66.

70. Wernli KJ, DeMartini WB, Ichikawa L, et al. Patterns of breast magnetic resonance imaging use in community practice. JAMA Intern Med 2014;174(1): 125–32.

71. Rahbar H, Hanna LG, Gatsonis C, et al. Contralateral prophylactic mastectomy in the American College of Radiology Imaging Network 6667 trial: effect of breast MR imaging assessments and patient characteristics. Radiology 2014;273(1):53–60.

72. Rahbar H, Lehmnan CD. Rethinking preoperative breast magnetic resonance imaging. JAMA Oncol 2015;1(9):1226–7.

73. Tuttle TM, Habermann EB, Grund EH, et al. Increasing use of contralateral prophylactic mastectomy for breast cancer patients: a trend toward more aggressive surgical treatment. J Clin Oncol 2007;25:5203–9.

74. Rosen PP. Invasive lobular carcinoma. Rosen's breast pathology. Philadelphia: Lippincott-Raven; 1997. p. 545–65.

75. Hilleren DJ, Andersson IT, Lindholm K, et al. Invasive lobular carcinoma: mammographic findings in a 10-year experience. Radiology 1991;178(1): 149–54.

76. Arpino G, Bardou VJ, Clark GM, et al. Infiltrating lobular carcinoma of the breast: tumor characteristics and clinical outcome. Breast Cancer Res 2004; 6(3):R149–56.

77. Keskek M, Kothari M, Ardehali B, et al. Factors predisposing to cavity margin positivity following conservation surgery for breast cancer. Eur J Surg Oncol 2004;30(10):1058–64.

78. O'Sullivan MJ, Li T, Freedman G, et al. The effect of multiple reexcisions on the risk of local recurrence after breast conserving surgery. Ann Surg Oncol 2007;14(11):3133–40.

79. Smitt MC, Horst K. Association of clinical and pathologic variables with lumpectomy surgical margin status after preoperative diagnosis or excisional biopsy of invasive breast cancer. Ann Surg Oncol 2007;14(3):1040–4.

80. van den Broek N, van der Sangen MJ, van de Poll-Franse LV, et al. Margin status and the risk of local recurrence after breast-conserving treatment of lobular breast cancer. Breast Cancer Res Treat 2007;105(1):63–8.

81. Waljee JF, Hu ES, Newman LA, et al. Predictors of re-excision among women undergoing breast-conserving surgery for cancer. Ann Surg Oncol 2008;15(5):1297–303.

82. Mann RM. The effectiveness of MR imaging in the assessment of invasive lobular carcinoma of the breast. Magn Reson Imaging Clin N Am 2010;18: 259–76.

83. Mann RM, Hoogeveen YL, Blickman JG, et al. MRI compared to conventional diagnostic work-up in the detection and evaluation of invasive lobular carcinoma of the breast: a review of existing literature. Breast Cancer Res Treat 2008;107(1):1–14.

84. Quan ML, Sclafani L, Heerdt AS, et al. Magnetic resonance imaging detects unsuspected disease in patients with invasive lobular cancer. Ann Surg Oncol 2003;10(9):1048–53.

85. Weinstein SP, Orel SG, Heller R, et al. MR imaging of the breast in patients with invasive lobular carcinoma. AJR Am J Roentgenol 2001;176(2):399–406.

86. Ernster VL, Barclay J, Kerlikowske K, et al. Mortality among women with ductal carcinoma in situ of the breast in the population-based surveillance, epidemiology and end results program. Arch Intern Med 2000;160:953–8.

87. Bijker N, Meijnen P, Peterse JL, et al. Breast-conserving treatment with or without radiotherapy in ductal-carcinoma-in situ: ten-year results of European Organisation for Research and Treatment of Cancer randomized phase III trial 10853—a study by the EORTC Breast Cancer Cooperative

Group and EORTC Radiotherapy Group. J Clin Oncol 2006;24:3381–7.

88. Silverstein MJ, Lagios MD, Groshen S, et al. The influence of margin width on local control of ductal carcinoma in situ of the breast. N Engl J Med 1999;340:1455–61.

89. MacDonald HR, Silverstein MJ, Lee LA, et al. Margin width as the sole determinant of local recurrence after breast conservation in patients with ductal carcinoma in situ of the breast. Am J Surg 2006;192:420–2.

90. Holland R, Conolly JL, Gelman R, et al. The presence of an extensive intraductal component following a limited excision correlates with prominent residual disease in the remainder of the breast. J Clin Oncol 1990;8:113–8.

91. Thomas J, Evans A, Macartney J, et al. Radiological and pathological size estimations of pure ductal carcinoma in situ of the breast, specimen handling and the influence on the success of breast conservation surgery: a review of 2564 cases from the Sloane Project. Br J Cancer 2010; 102:285–93.

92. Dillon MF, Mc Dermott EW, O'Doherty A, et al. Factors affecting successful breast conservation for ductal carcinoma in situ. Ann Surg Oncol 2007; 14(5):1618–28.

93. Berg WA, Gutierrez L, NessAvier MS, et al. Diagnostic accuracy of mammography, clinical examination US, and MR imaging in preoperative assessment of breast cancer. Radiology 2004; 233:830–49.

94. Hwang ES, Kinkel K, Esserman LJ, et al. Magnetic resonance imaging in patients diagnosed with ductal carcinoma-in-situ: value in the diagnosis of residual disease, occult invasion, and multicentricity. Ann Surg Oncol 2003;10(4):381–8.

95. Esserman LJ, Kumar AS, Herrera AF, et al. Magnetic resonance imaging captures the biology of ductal carcinoma in situ. J Clin Oncol 2006;24: 4603–10.

96. Marcotte-Bloch C, Balu-Maestro CB, Chamorey E, et al. MRI for the size assessment of pure ductal carcinoma in situ (DCIS): a prospective study of 33 patients. Eur J Radiol 2011;77(3):462–7.

97. Kuhl CK, Schrading S, Bieling HB, et al. MRI for diagnosis of pure ductal carcinoma in situ: a prospective observational study. Lancet 2007;370: 485–92.

98. Hollingsworth AB, Stough RG. Multicentric and contralateral invasive tumors identified with preop MRI in patients newly diagnosed with ductal carcinoma in situ of the breast. Breast J 2012; 18(5):420–7.

99. Allen LR, Lago-Toro CE, Hughes JH, et al. Is there a role for MRI in the preoperative assessment of patients with DCIS? Ann Surg Oncol 2010;17(9): 2395–400.

100. Kropcho LC, Steen ST, Chung AP, et al. Preoperative breast MRI in the surgical treatment of ductal carcinoma in situ. Breast J 2012;18:151–6.

101. Schouten van der Velden AP, Boetes C, Bult P, et al. The value of magnetic resonance imaging in diagnosis and size assessment of in situ and small invasive breast carcinoma. Am J Surg 2006;192:172–8.

102. Van Goethem M, Schelfout K, Kersschot E, et al. MR mammography is useful in the preoperative locoregional staging of breast carcinomas with extensive ductal component. Eur J Radiol 2007; 62:273–82.

103. Kumar AS, Chen DF, Au A, et al. Biologic significance of false-positive magnetic resonance imaging enhancement in the setting of ductal carcinoma in situ. Am J Surg 2006;192:520–4.

104. Fischer U, Zachariae O, Baum F, et al. The influence of preoperative MRI of the breasts on recurrence rate in patients with breast cancer. Eur Radiol 2004;14:1725–31.

105. Vapiwala N, Hwang WT, Kushner CJ, et al. No impact of breast magnetic resonance imaging on 15-year outcomes in patients with ductal carcinoma in situ or early-stage invasive breast cancer managed with breast conservation therapy. Cancer 2017;123:1324–32.

106. Gervais MK, Maki E, Schiller DE, et al. Preoperative MRI of the breast and ipsilateral breast tumor recurrence: long-term follow up. J Surg Oncol 2017;9999:1–7.

107. Nguyen PL, Taghian AG, Katz MS, et al. Breast cancer subtype approximated by estrogen receptor, progesterone receptor, and Her-2 is associated with local and distant recurrence after breast-conserving therapy. J Clin Oncol 2008;26: 2373–8.

108. Voduc KD, Cheang MC, Tyldesley S, et al. Breast cancer subtypes and the risk of local and regional relapse. J Clin Oncol 2010;28:1684–91.

109. Ha R, Jin B, Mango V, et al. Breast cancer molecular subtype as a predictor of the utility of preoperative MRI. AJR Am J Roentgenol 2015;204:1354–60.

Role of MR Imaging in Neoadjuvant Therapy Monitoring

Huong T. Le-Petross, MD[a],*, Bora Lim, MD[b]

KEYWORDS

- Breast cancer • Inflammatory breast cancer • Neoadjuvant chemotherapy
- Preoperative chemotherapy

KEY POINTS

- MR imaging is superior to physical examination and other imaging modalities in assessing neoadjuvant chemotherapy response and evaluating for residual disease before surgery.
- A combination of dynamic contrast-enhanced MR imaging and diffusion-weighted imaging provides better technique and promising tools for predicting response to neoadjuvant therapy, enabling early modification to therapy.
- MR imaging techniques remain variable, and standardization is needed.
- Changes in MR imaging features vary with different molecular subtypes of breast cancer.

INTRODUCTION

Breast cancer remains the most commonly diagnosed cancer in women.[1,2] Neoadjuvant or preoperative therapy has become an important treatment approach in stage II and III breast cancers. Traditional indications for neoadjuvant therapy in breast cancer include N2 stage, fixed or matted ipsilateral adenopathy, or clinically apparent ipsilateral internal mammary adenopathy in the absence of axillary adenopathy, making the clinical staging at least stage IIIA. Neoadjuvant chemotherapy (NAC) should also be considered for women with clinical stage IIA and IIB tumors with a larger tumor who wish avoid mastectomy and undergo breast-conserving surgery instead. In many patients, neoadjuvant therapy results in sufficient tumor response to make breast-conserving surgery possible. NAC can successfully reduce both breast tumor and local-regional nodal recurrence, even in large T3 and T4 tumors.[2,3] In one prospective study of 551 patients, the 5-year local-regional recurrence-free survival was similar between those who received mastectomy versus breast-conserving surgery.[3] More recently, pathologic complete remission is an important concept currently developed as a prognostic marker of survival in patients with breast cancer.[4,5] For human epidermal growth factor receptor 2 (HER2) overexpressing and triple-negative (TNBC) breast cancers, the pathologic response can also predict the long-term progression-free and overall survival rates.[4,5] In the current era of precision medicine, the importance of neoadjuvant therapy is even more critical and may serve as an investigation platform of new non–standard of care therapy. If responders can be distinguished from nonresponders early in the course of NAC, then early prediction on pathologic complete remission would give advantage to investigators who test their new drug or drugs in the neoadjuvant setting. MR imaging methods

The authors have nothing to disclose.
[a] Department of Diagnostic Imaging, University of Texas MD Anderson Cancer Center, 1155 Pressler Street, Houston, TX 77030, USA; [b] Department of Breast Medical Oncology, University of Texas MD Anderson Cancer Center, 1155 Pressler Street, Houston, TX 77030, USA
* Corresponding author.
E-mail address: hlepetross@mdanderson.org

Magn Reson Imaging Clin N Am 26 (2018) 207–220
https://doi.org/10.1016/j.mric.2017.12.011
1064-9689/18/Published by Elsevier Inc.

may be a valuable tool for providing this information while patients are on NAC.

ASSESSMENT OF RESPONSE BY CONVENTIONAL IMAGING

Historically, physical examination, mammography, and ultrasound have been used to assess response to NAC with limitations unique to each modality. Physical examination is unreliable and subjective, relying on the physician's experience, and is often difficult to separate residual tumor from posttreatment fibrosis or postbiopsy seroma. In one study, 45% of patients with normal physical examination had gross residual disease on pathology and 60% of patients with pathologic complete response (pCR) had an abnormal physical examination.[6] Physical examination had overestimated tumor regression in 23% of cases and underestimated response in 9%.[7]

Mammography is commonly used to assess response to therapy. Mammogram can overestimate residual disease due to background dense breast tissue obscuring true margins of residual tumor or a lack of change in the calcifications associated with the tumor after NAC (**Fig. 1**). A study of 196 patients with invasive ductal carcinoma and ductal carcinoma in situ (DCIS) reported that the extent of calcifications on mammography after NAC had lower correlation with residual pathologic tumor than did residual enhancement seen on MR imaging.[8] Even though ultrasound has been reported as being more accurate than physical examination and mammography, ultrasound tends to underestimate residual tumor size.[9–12] The posttreatment fibrosis is difficult to differentiate from residual viable tumor. As a result, the size estimation on imaging correlates only moderately with final pathologic tumor size.[12] The combination of mammography and ultrasound improves the imaging accuracy, with reported likelihood of pathologic complete response of 80%.[12] With additional investigation on contrast-enhanced ultrasound, a small sample size pilot study has suggested that contrast-enhanced ultrasound may be comparable to MR imaging.[13] Contrast-enhanced

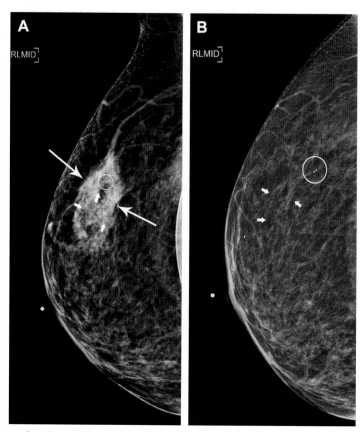

Fig. 1. Mammogram of a 47-year-old woman with a diagnosis of TNBC in the right breast. Pre-NAC lateral mammogram (*A*) revealed a 6-cm mass (*arrow*) and associated calcifications (*arrowheads*). Post-NAC lateral mammogram (*B*) revealed no residual mass but unchanged 8-cm area of calcifications (*arrowheads*). Biopsy clip denoted with circle in (*A*) and (*B*).

ultrasound would be a very attractive alternative for patients who have contraindications to having an MR imaging examination.

ASSESSMENT OF RESPONSE BY MR IMAGING

MR imaging was the first breast imaging modality requiring intravenous contrast that allows for not only detailed visualization of the anatomy but also enhancement characteristics of the tumor and surrounding tissue as well as detection of tumor angiogenesis. In addition to dynamic contrast-enhanced MR imaging (DCE-MR imaging), other MR imaging–specific techniques, such as diffusion-weighted (DWI) MR imaging, provides information on water proton mobility or Brownian motion without the need for intravenous contrast. This combination of DCE-MR imaging with DWI is better than either method alone because DCE-MR imaging provides higher specificity of 91% compared with 82% for DWI, whereas DWI provides higher sensitivity of 93% compared with 68% for DCE-MR imaging, as reported in 2 meta-analyses of up to 54 studies.[14,15] New MR imaging sequence exploration and development are ongoing to find the optimal sequence or sequences or combination of sequences for predicting response in patients, with the goal of identifying those patients who would benefit from modification to their NAC regimens. Several newer non–MR imaging modalities, such as PET/computed tomography (CT) and molecular breast imaging, are also being evaluated to determine their performance and role in assessing response to therapy. Currently, there is still a lack of published data supporting the use of one imaging modality or technique over another, and no guidelines for imaging modality or regimen to be used in assessing response during therapy. Preliminary data from observational studies suggest that PET/CT performs better than breast MR imaging in hormone-positive/HER2-negative and TNBC subtypes.[14] This article reviews only the published data on the role of breast MR imaging in assessing tumor response in women receiving NAC.

MR IMAGING PROTOCOL

In most centers in the United States, MR imaging sequences used for assessing response to therapy are similar if not identical to breast MR imaging examinations performed for other indications, such as screening high-risk patients or for staging newly diagnosed breast cancer. This standard MR imaging examination usually consists of precontrast T1-weighted series, T2-weighted/bright fluid

series, multiphase T1-weighted series with precontrast, and 3 or more postcontrast series.[16] Breast MR imaging examinations have been performed on a 0.5-T, 1-T, 1.5-T, or 3-T magnetic system, with 1.5 T and 3 T being the most common. In addition, some centers are now performing routine DWI sequences either before or after intravenous contrast administration. Investigators have looked at using only one sequence such as T2 relaxation times to determine if this parameter can reflect the underlying biological state of the tumor. It was observed that the lesion T2 relaxation time was reduced (64.50 ms) after NAC compared with before NAC (81.34 ms), and this measurement was also shorter with responders (63.18 ms) than nonresponders (74.62 ms).[17] Tumor heterogeneity on T2-weighted sequences was different between responders and nonresponders as well as different between the baseline or pre-NAC MR imaging and the mid-therapy MR imaging.[18] It was suggested that a noncontrast sequence such as T2-weighted may better reflect the underlying biological tumor change from NAC than DCE-MR imaging because the contrast agent distribution and vascular features on contrast images can mask underlying morphologic changes not associated with vascularity.[17,18]

RESPONSE ASSESSMENT USING MR IMAGING SIZE

The shifting from systemic adjuvant therapy to neoadjuvant therapy in the last decade offers several benefits, including an accelerated evaluation of new drugs or combination of drugs. Clinical trials still use tumor size change to determine response. Therefore, accurate tumor size measurement is important during and after NAC for assessing midtherapy response as well as providing information on residual tumor burden prior to surgery. MR imaging more accurately reflects true pathologic tumor size than physical examination, mammography, or ultrasound in predicting the amount of residual disease after NAC.[19–22] MR imaging may still underestimate in approximately 10% of cases and overestimate final tumor size in up to 33% of cases, but only within 1 cm of the final tumor size when compared with gross histology,[23,24] with reported correlation coefficient ranging between 0.6 and 0.9.[25–27]

Tumor volume calculations, in place of or in combination with largest tumor diameter, have been observed as having a stronger association with recurrence-free survival than other prognostic indicators. This volume change can be observed as early as after one cycle of chemotherapy[28]

(Fig. 2). The American College of Radiology Imaging Network 6657/Investigation of Serial Studies to Predict Your Therapeutic Response with Imaging and Molecular Analysis (I-SPY) trial showed that tumor volume was a better predictor of response than change in the largest diameter, and the volume change had the greatest benefit at the second MR examination or after one cycle of anthracycline-based treatment.[28] Adaptive response clinical trials, such as the I-SPY trial, involve the "adaptive statistical design" of breast cancer, selecting the next best alternative targeted therapy based on the response to the systemic therapy. Therefore, accurate response assessment is critical in the care of the patient. Ultrasound is still more widely used for image-based monitoring of response, even though MR imaging would be the better imaging modality to assess intermediate treatment response while the novel therapy is ongoing or to guide decision making with regards to patient allocation into the adaptive trial.

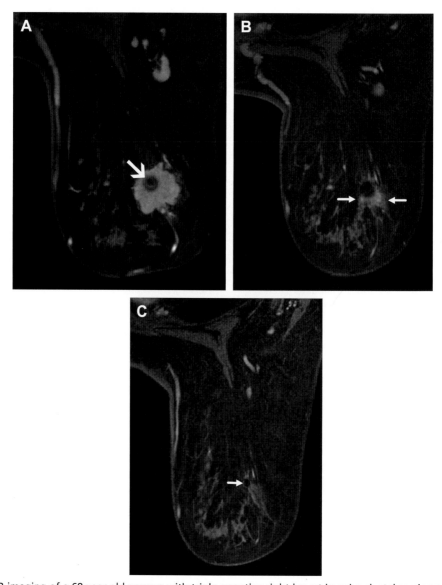

Fig. 2. MR imaging of a 68-year-old woman with triple-negative right breast invasive ductal carcinoma. (A) Pre-NAC axial postcontrast MR image showing the irregular 3-cm biopsy-proven carcinoma with an associated biopsy clip (arrow). (B) Second MR image after one cycle of anthracycline-based therapy showed decreased in size of tumor mass (arrows). (C) Post-NAC MR image shows no residual enhancing mass at the site of the biopsy clip (arrow), compatible with complete imaging response to therapy. Final pathology confirmed complete response.

RESPONSE ASSESSMENT USING MR IMAGING MORPHOLOGY

Defining the margins of the breast tumors in order to accurately measure the largest diameter or calculate the tumor volume can be challenging during and after NAC.[27] Tumors may present as a dominant mass, multiple masses, and/or non–mass enhancement (**Fig. 3**). MR imaging is accurate for assessing mass lesions that have clear margins for measurement or that enhances more than the background parenchyma. Tumors that present as masses also tend to shrink to smaller masses or nodules, allowing for accurate size measurement.[29] Non–mass-enhancement lesions (classically representing invasive lobular carcinoma or DCIS), are detectable with MR imaging, but accurate size measurement can be a challenge with any imaging modality. These lesions tend to break up into small islands of tumor or become fragmented during therapy (**Fig. 4**). The residual disease may be scattered cells or even single cell in the background of posttreatment fibrosis, making it difficult to measure the size of the residual disease. In these cases, MR imaging is likely to underestimate residual disease in up to 10% of cases, where the tumor shrinkage pattern is patchy with areas of fibrosis between nests of viable tumor or tiny tumor foci scattered over a large area.[23,30,31] The pattern of tumor regression is also observed to be different between the various subtypes of breast cancer. One study categorized tumor shrinkage pattern as being in a concentric pattern without surrounding lesions, concentric pattern with surrounding lesions, residual multinodular lesions, or whole quadrant diffuse residual enhancement.[32]

The breast cancer molecular subtypes include the luminal A (hormonal positive, HER2-negative), luminal B (hormonal positive, HER2-positive), triple negative or basal-like, and HER-positive cancers. There is limited data on the use of MR imaging for assessing response

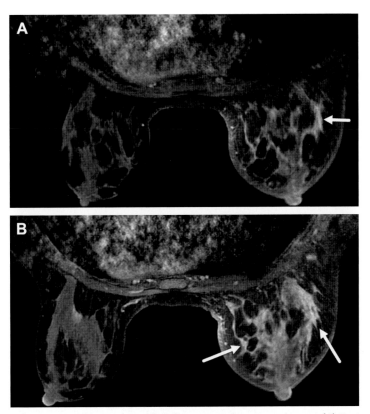

Fig. 3. MR imaging of a 27-year-old woman with inflammatory breast carcinoma. (*A*) Post–contrast-enhanced T1-weighted image revealed diffuse breast enlargement with global skin thickening and non–mass enhancement throughout the breast parenchyma. Biopsy-proven high-grade DCIS with microinvasive carcinoma was performed of an area in the lateral breast (*arrow*). (*B*) Post–contrast-enhanced T1-weighted image revealed global increased breast enlargement and non–mass enhancement (*arrows*) with global skin thickening, consistent with disease progression while on NAC.

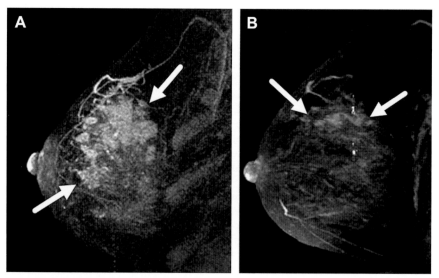

Fig. 4. MR imaging of a 28-year-old woman with HER2-positive invasive ductal carcinoma. (*A*) Maximum intensity projection image shows multiple small masses and non–mass enhancement predominantly in the superior and central right breast (*arrows*). (*B*) After NAC, there is residual non–mass enhancement that is difficult to measure with an estimated size of 4 cm (*arrows*). Final pathology at mastectomy revealed 0.4-cm invasive carcinoma, 3 cm of residual DCIS, and dense stromal fibrosis consistent with posttreatment changes.

to NAC in hormone receptor–positive breast cancer (**Fig. 5**). This is partly related to the fact that the benefit of NAC in this subtype remains unclear. The European Organization for Research and Treatment of Cancer trial 10902 compared the outcome of NAC versus adjuvant chemotherapy. The progression-free survival, overall survival, and local recurrence rates were not different between NAC and conventional postoperative chemotherapy.[33] In a study of 250 patients, MR imaging size correlation was significantly better with estrogen receptor (ER)-negative tumors ($r = 0.76$) than ER-positive tumors ($r = 0.40$).[34] MR imaging was observed to be of limited benefit in predicting pCR in ER-positive tumors.[14] FDG-PET/CT performed better than MR imaging for hormone receptor–positive/HER2-negative breast cancer.[14] For TNBC, both FDG-PET/CT and MR imaging seem promising as diagnostic tools for assessing response.[14] TNBCs are usually larger, more defined masses, and more likely to be necrotic, which make them easier to visualize and measure.[35] MR imaging performed after 2 NAC cycles to detect size reduction showed correlation with pathology. The decrease in largest diameter of late enhancement showed significant association with tumor regression.[36] The presence of central or intratumoral necrosis is associated with poor response.[37,38] For HER2-positive breast cancer, HER2 therapy is very effective in reducing the tumor size. Concentric shrinkage

was associated with Her2-positive breast cancer.[32] Tumor size reduction, defined as a change in the largest diameter of late enhancement seen between the MR imaging examinations performed before and during NAC, was associated with response to therapy.[36]

Breast cancer is a complex heterogeneous disease as confirmed with texture analysis, which measures the tumor heterogeneity based on statistical modeling. Changes in texture could be observed on T2-weighted or contrast-enhanced dynamic series. Within a tumor, there are subregions that have distinct enhancement, and the heterogeneity of the internal enhancement patterns between the subregions may directly or indirectly reflect underlying growth pattern, which may prove useful in assessing response.[39]

RESPONSE ASSESSMENT USING MR IMAGING KINETICS

The role of MR imaging kinetics regarding its usefulness in predicting response remains unclear. The increase or decrease in enhancement seen during or after NAC may correlate with response. Tumor enhancement is characterized as very early phase (0–60 seconds), initial enhancement (60–120 seconds) of the dynamic series, or delayed phase (more than 120 seconds) after injection of a gadolinium-based intravenous contrast. Aggressive tumors are more likely to

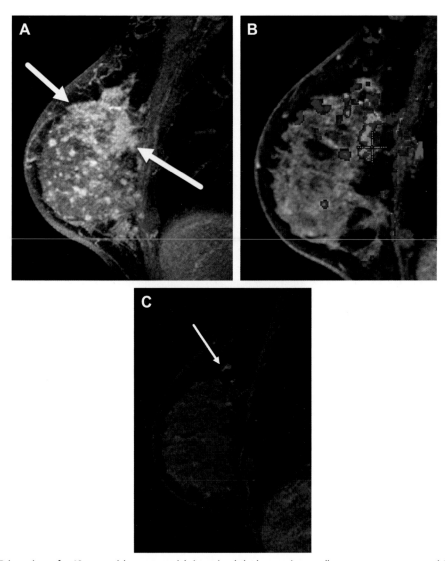

Fig. 5. MR imaging of a 49-year-old woman with invasive lobular carcinoma (hormone receptor–positive, HER2-negative) who received NAC followed by mastectomy. (A) Pre-NAC MR imaging showed a 4.3-cm area of non–mass enhancement (arrows) in the upper breast corresponding to site of biopsy-proven carcinoma. (B) Colorized map shows heterogeneous enhancement with the red color showing foci with delayed washout kinetic curve. (C) Post-NAC MR imaging shows no residual enhancement at the tumor bed (arrow), suggesting complete response. Final pathology revealed residual invasive lobular carcinoma with therapy effect extending over an area of 10 cm in all quadrants, 15% cellularity. MR imaging markedly underestimated residual disease and does not perform as well with hormone receptor positive or HER2 negative as with TNBC or HER2-positive cancer.

display a greater degree of angiogenesis, demonstrate as high vascular perfusion and permeability, and are associated with worse prognosis.[40,41] Theoretically, the pharmacokinetic parameters should be helpful in predicting response, but this has not been consistently observed. Some of the kinetic changes associated with complete histologic response include the disappearance or normalization of the early or initial abnormal enhancement,[19] flattening of the time-intensity curve, disappearance of the delayed washout curve after one course of chemotherapy, or the absence of enhancement at the tumor bed after 4 courses of chemotherapy[42] (Fig. 6). The decrease in both the rate and magnitude of contrast enhancement within the tumor mass versus an increase or no change was also found to correlate with responders versus nonresponders, respectively.[43,44] The dynamic contrast-enhanced kinetics is usually

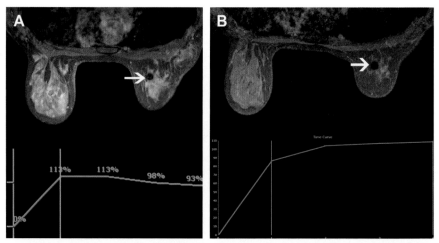

Fig. 6. MR imaging of a 49-year-old woman with invasive lobular carcinoma (hormone receptor–positive, HER2-negative) who received NAC followed by mastectomy. MR imaging kinetics of the tumor shows delayed washout before NAC (*A*). After 2 cycles of NAC, the tumor demonstrates delayed persistent kinetic curve (*B*). Arrow denotes biopsy clip in (*A*) and (*B*).

measured manually by placing a region of interest (ROI) in an area of the enhancing tumor bed, and the most suspicious kinetic curve within the ROI is reported. This technique is associated with variability in measurement. Further analysis of the vascular properties of breast tumor by vascular parameters, such as the forward volume transfer constant (K^{trans}) and the reverse transvascular transfer rate constant (k_{ep}), did not improve prediction of early response compared with size change.[45] A host of factors, including variability in reported data due to differences in sample size, tumor subtypes, chemotherapy agents, and analytical techniques, make it difficult to compare the various studies. The combination of changes in overall tumor volume and voxel analysis of contrast enhancement time curves may improve the specificity of diagnosis and produce clinically meaningful information about tumor heterogeneity, permeability, and vascularity.

RESPONSE ASSESSMENT USING OTHER MR IMAGING FEATURES

Edema is well seen on MR imaging, presenting as high signal intensity on T2-weighted images. For breast cancer cases with edema, bright T2-weighted signals can be seen in the subcutaneous tissue, around the tumor bed, or in the prepectoral location (**Fig. 7**). Prepectoral edema is commonly seen with large tumor size, higher grade tumor,

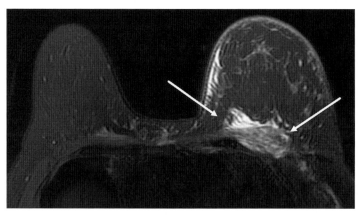

Fig. 7. MR imaging of a 77-year-old woman with inflammatory invasive ductal breast carcinoma. Non–contrast-enhanced T2-weighted image of the enlarged left breast showing prepectoral and pectoral edema with diffuse increased signal intensity (*arrows*).

greater lymphovascular invasion, and inflammatory breast cancer (IBC).[46] Prepectoral edema was not identified in any of the 129 benign lesions but seen in 9% of the breast cancers (460/589).[46] However, edema can occur with nonmalignant conditions as well. The resolution of this edema has not been reported to be a biomarker for detection of early response.

DWI assesses water molecule and is an unenhanced MR imaging technique that provides information on microscopic water proton mobility known as Brownian motion. This motion is sensitive to cell or tissue density and membrane integrity.[47] The apparent diffusion coefficient (ADC) is a quantitative derivative that has demonstrated promise as an early surrogate biopsy biomarker for detecting early response to therapy. Tumors generally have high density, and therefore, low ADC value. After NAC, tumors that respond would have decreased cell density with increase extracellular space, and as a result, higher ADC value than before treatment.[48,49] This is observed in patients undergoing NAC, with statistically significantly lower ADC values before treatment than after treatment in responders.[41,46,49] Furthermore, the mean percentage ADC increase in responders (47.9%) was higher than that in nonresponders (18.1%) (P<.001).[50] This mean percentage change in ADC was statistically significant between clinical responders compared with nonresponders, whereas the changes in volume and diameter were not significantly different between responders and nonresponders.[49] Sensitivity of DWI was 93% and specificity was 82% in a meta-analysis.[51] The combination of DWI and DCE-MR imaging is superior to each technique alone.[52] Other combinations of DWI with PET/CT showed a 54.9% increase in the ADC and a 63.9% decrease in the standardized uptake value as the best cutoff to differentiate responders from nonresponders, with sensitivity reaching up to 100% and specificity of 70.4%.[53]

The use of DWI to visualize residual disease without the need of intravenous contrast sounds appealing, and yet this technique is still not widely accepted as standard technique to assess response. This lack of widespread use may be due to the limitations of DWI methods. One limitation is the lower spatial resolution of DWI compared with DCE-MR imaging. Without the corresponding DCE-MR images for correlation, a residual small tumor may not be detectable on DWI. The methodologic differences in ROI measurements, b-value, ADC cutoff values, and fat suppression techniques are quite variable between publications, and standardization is needed for this to be widely used and compared between

treatment protocols. Non–mass lesions and non–mass enhancement are more challenging, and DWI may not be able to predict response as observed with mass lesions.[54]

RESPONSE ASSESSMENT USING MR IMAGING BY BREAST CANCER SUBTYPE

The accuracy of MR imaging in estimating residual disease after NAC is affected by the subtype of breast cancer.[14,32,36,55] Hormonal status such as estrogen receptor and progesterone receptor affects the response to chemotherapy, and consequently, the accuracy of post-NAC MR imaging. MR imaging seems more accurate in HER2-positive and TNBC cancers and can predict pCR after 2 cycles of chemotherapy.[55] Sensitivity was reported at 93.1%.[55] The reported negative predictive value of 60% is also highest for patients with hormone receptor–negative and HER2-positive breast cancer, as observed in a multicenter study of 746 patients.[56] Targeted therapy, such as trastuzumab, against HER2-positive cancer is very effective. In NAC cases showing complete (or near complete) pCR, there is less likelihood of residual scattered disease confounding the accuracy of MR imaging, because MR imaging has limited accuracy in detecting residual disease that is small foci, scattered cells, or small cell clusters.[29,57] MR imaging would be expected to perform better with HER2-positive cancer than HER2-negative cancers.

RESPONSE ASSESSMENT USING MR IMAGING IN INFLAMMATORY BREAST CANCER

IBC is a rare but advanced type of breast cancer.[58] The diagnosis of IBC is a clinical (and not imaging) diagnosis, with a combination of the following symptoms presenting rapidly within a few weeks or few months: breast erythema, breast edema, "peau d'orange" skin changes with or without an underlying palpable mass, tenderness, and/or diffuseness of tumor by palpation. Despite increased awareness of diagnosis among physicians and patients, challenges remain in various aspects of IBC diagnosis and treatment. Current imaging assessment includes mammogram, ultrasound with possible biopsy of a breast lesion and metastatic node, breast MR imaging, and PET/CT (**Fig. 8**). MR imaging can detect a primary breast lesion in 98% of the cases, and the most common finding was an index mass or multiple small masses (73%). The skin abnormalities, such as skin thickening, skin edema, and skin nodules or enhancing

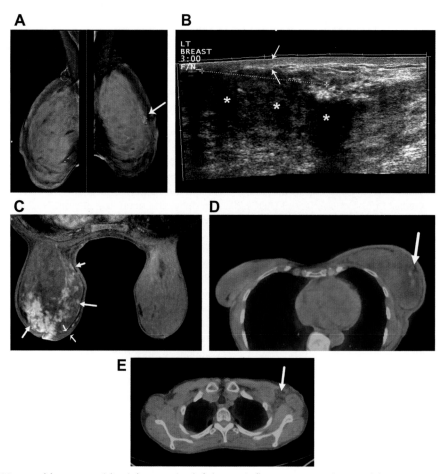

Fig. 8. A 66-year-old woman with triple-negative left breast inflammatory carcinoma. (*A*) Mammogram showed dense breast tissue bilaterally with suspicious 2-cm area of calcifications in the left breast (*arrow*). (*B*) Ultrasound showed a 4-cm area of abnormal hypoechoic tissue (*asterisks*), compatible with the biopsy-proven carcinoma, and diffuse skin thickening (*arrows*). (*C*) MR imaging showed multiple enhancing masses and non–mass enhancement with multicentric distribution involving all 4 quadrants (*thick arrows*), along with diffuse skin thickening (*thin arrows*). (*D*) PET/CT showed hypermetabolic lesions primarily in the lateral left breast (*arrow*). (*E*) PET/CT showed left axillary adenopathy (*arrow*).

foci, are also best detected with MR imaging than other modality, such as ultrasound and mammography. Because the disease is best seen with MR imaging, response prediction and residual tumor size correlation with final pathology are also better with MR imaging than ultrasound or mammography.[59] When a primary breast lesion can be identified, the kinetic enhancing curve is most commonly rapid initial enhancement with delayed washout enhancing pattern (type III) as expected for patients with non-IBC cancer. The enhancement is more commonly type I persistent enhancing pattern in patients who respond to NAC. A study of 47 patients with locally advanced breast cancer and 13 patients with IBC, using RNA microarray and DCE-MR imaging, found an association between the DCE-MR imaging perfusion pattern and gene expression profiles.[60] The literature on this is limited due to the rarity of the disease. IBC tends to show more nodal metastases (77.8%) and distant metastases (39.7%) compared with non-IBC locally advanced breast cancer (nodal metastases 69.7% and distant metastases 34.1%)[33] (**Fig. 9**). Therefore, the treatment of IBC is slightly different compared with non-IBC breast cancers. Early diagnosis, aggressive NAC, mastectomy, and adjuvant radiotherapy, combined with continued development of targeted therapy, are the key to achieving the best clinical outcome for IBC patients.

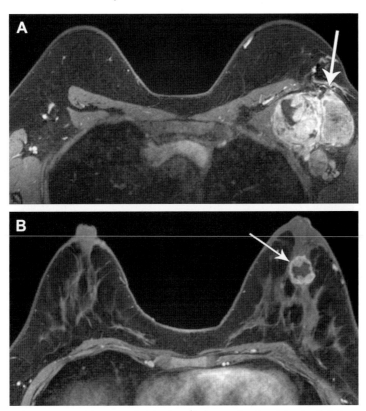

Fig. 9. MR imaging of a 33-year-old woman with clinical diagnosis of IBC in the left breast. (*A*) Postcontrast gradient echo axial image shows extensive left axillary adenopathy with perinodal edema or stranding (*arrow*). (*B*) Postcontrast dynamic series revealed a centrally necrotic left breast mass (*arrow*), and biopsy confirmed invasive ductal carcinoma.

SUMMARY

Multimodality treatment of breast cancer has improved survival and reduced the risk of recurrence.[61] NAC has been shown to convert unresectable cancers to resectable cancers, allowing for breast-conserving surgery in these patients, with equivalent rates of disease-free survival and overall survival when compared with adjuvant chemotherapy.[62] Numerous single-center trials from several countries examining the role of breast MR imaging in monitoring tumor response to NAC have shown that MR imaging correlates better with residual disease seen on final pathology than does mammography or ultrasound. Some MR imaging features allow for earlier prediction of response to therapy, relative to mammography or ultrasound. The combination of DCE-MR imaging and DWI appears to be the best imaging modality currently, because there are limited data on PET-MR imaging combination. Comparison of the published data is difficult due to differences in MR imaging scanners, definition of response, chemotherapy agents, and chemotherapy regimens. Most studies were single-center trials with a relatively small sample size. More recent publications address the imaging findings and response based on biomarker profile of the primary breast cancer in the current era of personalized medicine and increasingly individualized therapy regimens. For MR imaging to be more widely used, there needs to be standardization of MR imaging techniques such as b-values for DWI, combination of techniques of DCE-MR imaging with one or more of the functional imaging MR imaging techniques to improve the accuracy and minimize the false negative rate in the assessment of residual disease after NAC.

REFERENCES

1. Siegel RL, Miller KD, Jemal A. Cancer statistics, 2016. CA Cancer J Clin 2016;66(1):7–30.
2. Sweeting RS, Klauber-Demore N, Meyers MO, et al. Young women with locally advanced breast cancer who achieve breast conservation after neoadjuvant chemotherapy have a low local recurrence rate. Am Surg 2011;77(7):850–5.
3. Akay CL, Meric-Bernstam F, Hunt KK, et al. Evaluation of the MD Anderson Prognostic Index for

local-regional recurrence after breast conserving therapy in patients receiving neoadjuvant chemotherapy. Ann Surg Oncol 2012;19(3):901–7.

4. von Minckwitz G, Untch M, Blohmer JU, et al. Definition and impact of pathologic complete response on prognosis after neoadjuvant chemotherapy in various intrinsic breast cancer subtypes. J Clin Oncol 2012;30(15):1796–804.

5. Matuschek C, Bolke E, Roth SL, et al. Long-term outcome after neoadjuvant radiochemotherapy in locally advanced noninflammatory breast cancer and predictive factors for a pathologic complete remission: results of a multivariate analysis. Strahlenther Onkol 2012;188(9):777–81.

6. Feldman LD, Hortobagyi GN, Buzdar AU, et al. Pathological assessment of response to induction chemotherapy in breast cancer. Cancer Res 1986; 46(5):2578–81.

7. Cocconi G, Di Blasio B, Alberti G, et al. Problems in evaluating response of primary breast cancer to systemic therapy. Breast Cancer Res Treat 1984; 4(4):309–13.

8. Prati R, Minami CA, Gornbein JA, et al. Accuracy of clinical evaluation of locally advanced breast cancer in patients receiving neoadjuvant chemotherapy. Cancer 2009;115(6):1194–202.

9. Keune JD, Jeffe DB, Schootman M, et al. Accuracy of ultrasonography and mammography in predicting pathologic response after neoadjuvant chemotherapy for breast cancer. Am J Surg 2010;199(4):477–84.

10. Finlayson CA, MacDermott TA. Ultrasound can estimate the pathologic size of infiltrating ductal carcinoma. Arch Surg 2000;135(2):158–9.

11. Herrada J, Iyer RB, Atkinson EN, et al. Relative value of physical examination, mammography, and breast sonography in evaluating the size of the primary tumor and regional lymph node metastases in women receiving neoadjuvant chemotherapy for locally advanced breast carcinoma. Clin Cancer Res 1997;3(9):1565–9.

12. Chagpar AB, Middleton LP, Sahin AA, et al. Accuracy of physical examination, ultrasonography, and mammography in predicting residual pathologic tumor size in patients treated with neoadjuvant chemotherapy. Ann Surg 2006;243(2):257–64.

13. Lee SC, Grant E, Sheth P, et al. Accuracy of contrast-enhanced ultrasound compared with magnetic resonance imaging in assessing the tumor response after neoadjuvant chemotherapy for breast cancer. J Ultrasound Med 2017;36(5):901–11.

14. Lindenberg MA, Miquel-Cases A, Retel VP, et al. Imaging performance in guiding response to neoadjuvant therapy according to breast cancer subtypes: a systematic literature review. Crit Rev Oncol Hematol 2017;112:198–207.

15. Gu YL, Pan SM, Ren J, et al. Role of magnetic resonance imaging in detection of pathologic complete remission in breast cancer patients treated with neoadjuvant chemotherapy: a meta-analysis. Clin Breast Cancer 2017. https://doi.org/10.1016/j.clbc.2016.12.010.

16. Moy L, Newell MS, Mahoney MC, et al. ACR appropriateness criteria stage I breast cancer: initial workup and surveillance for local recurrence and distant metastases in asymptomatic women. J Am Coll Radiol 2016;13(11S):e43–52.

17. Liu L, Yin B, Geng DY, et al. Changes of T2 relaxation time from neoadjuvant chemotherapy in breast cancer lesions. Iran J Radiol 2016;13(3):e24014.

18. Henderson S, Purdie C, Michie C, et al. Interim heterogeneity changes measured using entropy texture features on T2-weighted MRI at 3.0 T are associated with pathological response to neoadjuvant chemotherapy in primary breast cancer. Eur Radiol 2017. https://doi.org/10.1007/s00330-017-4850-8.

19. Balu-Maestro C, Chapellier C, Bleuse A, et al. Imaging in evaluation of response to neoadjuvant breast cancer treatment benefits of MRI. Breast Cancer Res Treat 2002;72(2):145–52.

20. Cheung YC, Chen SC, Su MY, et al. Monitoring the size and response of locally advanced breast cancers to neoadjuvant chemotherapy (weekly paclitaxel and epirubicin) with serial enhanced MRI. Breast Cancer Res Treat 2003;78(1):51–8.

21. Gilles R, Guinebretiere JM, Toussaint C, et al. Locally advanced breast cancer: contrast-enhanced subtraction MR imaging of response to preoperative chemotherapy. Radiology 1994;191(3):633–8.

22. Yeh E, Slanetz P, Kopans DB, et al. Prospective comparison of mammography, sonography, and MRI in patients undergoing neoadjuvant chemotherapy for palpable breast cancer. AJR Am J Roentgenol 2005;184(3):868–77.

23. Rosen EL, Blackwell KL, Baker JA, et al. Accuracy of MRI in the detection of residual breast cancer after neoadjuvant chemotherapy. AJR Am J Roentgenol 2003;181(5):1275–82.

24. Lorenzon M, Zuiani C, Londero V, et al. Assessment of breast cancer response to neoadjuvant chemotherapy: is volumetric MRI a reliable tool? Eur J Radiol 2009;71(1):82–8.

25. Akazawa K, Tamaki Y, Taguchi T, et al. Preoperative evaluation of residual tumor extent by three-dimensional magnetic resonance imaging in breast cancer patients treated with neoadjuvant chemotherapy. Breast J 2006;12(2):130–7.

26. Belli P, Costantini M, Malaspina C, et al. MRI accuracy in residual disease evaluation in breast cancer patients treated with neoadjuvant chemotherapy. Clin Radiol 2006;61(11):946–53.

27. Partridge SC, Gibbs JE, Lu Y, et al. MRI measurements of breast tumor volume predict response to

neoadjuvant chemotherapy and recurrence-free survival. AJR Am J Roentgenol 2005;184(6):1774–81.

28. Hylton NM, Blume JD, Bernreuter WK, et al. Locally advanced breast cancer: MR imaging for prediction of response to neoadjuvant chemotherapy–results from ACRIN 6657/I-SPY TRIAL. Radiology 2012; 263(3):663–72.

29. Bahri S, Chen JH, Mehta RS, et al. Residual breast cancer diagnosed by MRI in patients receiving neoadjuvant chemotherapy with and without bevacizumab. Ann Surg Oncol 2009; 16(6):1619–28.

30. Wasser K, Sinn HP, Fink C, et al. Accuracy of tumor size measurement in breast cancer using MRI is influenced by histological regression induced by neoadjuvant chemotherapy. Eur Radiol 2003;13(6): 1213–23.

31. Warren RM, Bobrow LG, Earl HM, et al. Can breast MRI help in the management of women with breast cancer treated by neoadjuvant chemotherapy? Br J Cancer 2004;90(7):1349–60.

32. Ballesio L, Gigli S, Di Pastena F, et al. Magnetic resonance imaging tumor regression shrinkage patterns after neoadjuvant chemotherapy in patients with locally advanced breast cancer: correlation with tumor biological subtypes and pathological response after therapy. Tumour Biol 2017;39(3). 1010428317694540.

33. van der Hage JA, van de Velde CJ, Julien JP, et al. Preoperative chemotherapy in primary operable breast cancer: results from the European Organization for Research and Treatment of Cancer trial 10902. J Clin Oncol 2001;19(22): 4224–37.

34. Charehbili A, Wasser MN, Smit VT, et al. Accuracy of MRI for treatment response assessment after taxane- and anthracycline-based neoadjuvant chemotherapy in HER2-negative breast cancer. Eur J Surg Oncol 2014;40(10):1216–21.

35. Youk JH, Son EJ, Chung J, et al. Triple-negative invasive breast cancer on dynamic contrast-enhanced and diffusion-weighted MR imaging: comparison with other breast cancer subtypes. Eur Radiol 2012;22(8):1724–34.

36. Loo CE, Straver ME, Rodenhuis S, et al. Magnetic resonance imaging response monitoring of breast cancer during neoadjuvant chemotherapy: relevance of breast cancer subtype. J Clin Oncol 2011;29(6): 660–6.

37. Lee HJ, Song IH, Seo AN, et al. Correlations between molecular subtypes and pathologic response patterns of breast cancers after neoadjuvant chemotherapy. Ann Surg Oncol 2015;22(2): 392–400.

38. Kawashima H, Inokuchi M, Furukawa H, et al. Magnetic resonance imaging features of breast cancer according to intrinsic subtypes: correlations with neoadjuvant chemotherapy effects. Springerplus 2014;3:240.

39. Waugh SA, Purdie CA, Jordan LB, et al. Magnetic resonance imaging texture analysis classification of primary breast cancer. Eur Radiol 2016;26(2): 322–30.

40. Pickles MD, Manton DJ, Lowry M, et al. Prognostic value of pre-treatment DCE-MRI parameters in predicting disease free and overall survival for breast cancer patients undergoing neoadjuvant chemotherapy. Eur J Radiol 2009;71(3):498–505.

41. Ah-See ML, Makris A, Taylor NJ, et al. Early changes in functional dynamic magnetic resonance imaging predict for pathologic response to neoadjuvant chemotherapy in primary breast cancer. Clin Cancer Res 2008;14(20):6580–9.

42. Martincich L, Montemurro F, De Rosa G, et al. Monitoring response to primary chemotherapy in breast cancer using dynamic contrast-enhanced magnetic resonance imaging. Breast Cancer Res Treat 2004; 83(1):67–76.

43. Rieber A, Brambs HJ, Gabelmann A, et al. Breast MRI for monitoring response of primary breast cancer to neo-adjuvant chemotherapy. Eur Radiol 2002; 12(7):1711–9.

44. Kim HJ, Im YH, Han BK, et al. Accuracy of MRI for estimating residual tumor size after neoadjuvant chemotherapy in locally advanced breast cancer: relation to response patterns on MRI. Acta Oncol 2007;46(7):996–1003.

45. Yu HJ, Chen JH, Mehta RS, et al. MRI measurements of tumor size and pharmacokinetic parameters as early predictors of response in breast cancer patients undergoing neoadjuvant anthracycline chemotherapy. J Magn Reson Imaging 2007; 26(3):615–23.

46. Uematsu T, Kasami M, Watanabe J. Is evaluation of the presence of prepectoral edema on T2-weighted with fat-suppression 3 T breast MRI a simple and readily available noninvasive technique for estimation of prognosis in patients with breast cancer? Breast Cancer 2014;21(6):684–92.

47. O'Flynn EA, DeSouza NM. Functional magnetic resonance: biomarkers of response in breast cancer. Breast Cancer Res 2011;13(1):204.

48. Pickles MD, Gibbs P, Lowry M, et al. Diffusion changes precede size reduction in neoadjuvant treatment of breast cancer. Magn Reson Imaging 2006;24(7):843–7.

49. Sharma U, Danishad KK, Seenu V, et al. Longitudinal study of the assessment by MRI and diffusion-weighted imaging of tumor response in patients with locally advanced breast cancer undergoing neoadjuvant chemotherapy. NMR Biomed 2009; 22(1):104–13.

50. Park SH, Moon WK, Cho N, et al. Diffusion-weighted MR imaging: pretreatment prediction of response to

neoadjuvant chemotherapy in patients with breast cancer. Radiology 2010;257(1):56–63.

51. Wu LM, Hu J, Gu HY, et al. Can diffusion-weighted magnetic resonance imaging (DW-MRI) alone be used as a reliable sequence for the preoperative detection and characterisation of hepatic metastases? A meta-analysis. Eur J Cancer 2013;49(3): 572–84.

52. Belli P, Costantini M, Ierardi C, et al. Diffusion-weighted imaging in evaluating the response to neoadjuvant breast cancer treatment. Breast J 2011; 17(6):610–9.

53. Park SH, Moon WK, Cho N, et al. Comparison of diffusion-weighted MR imaging and FDG PET/CT to predict pathological complete response to neoadjuvant chemotherapy in patients with breast cancer. Eur Radiol 2012;22(1):18–25.

54. Kawamura M, Satake H, Ishigaki S, et al. Early prediction of response to neoadjuvant chemotherapy for locally advanced breast cancer using MRI. Nagoya J Med Sci 2011;73(3–4):147–56.

55. Fatayer H, Sharma N, Manuel D, et al. Serial MRI scans help in assessing early response to neoadjuvant chemotherapy and tailoring breast cancer treatment. Eur J Surg Oncol 2016;42(7):965–72.

56. De Los Santos JF, Cantor A, Amos KD, et al. Magnetic resonance imaging as a predictor of pathologic response in patients treated with neoadjuvant

systemic treatment for operable breast cancer. Translational Breast Cancer Research Consortium trial 017. Cancer 2013;119(10):1776–83.

57. Chen JH, Feig B, Agrawal G, et al. MRI evaluation of pathologically complete response and residual tumors in breast cancer after neoadjuvant chemotherapy. Cancer 2008;112(1):17–26.

58. Lu J, Steeg PS, Price JE, et al. Breast cancer metastasis: challenges and opportunities. Cancer Res 2009;69(12):4951–3.

59. Shin HJ, Kim HH, Ahn JH, et al. Comparison of mammography, sonography, MRI and clinical examination in patients with locally advanced or inflammatory breast cancer who underwent neoadjuvant chemotherapy. Br J Radiol 2011;84(1003):612–20.

60. Siamakpour-Reihani S, Owzar K, Jiang C, et al. Genomic profiling in locally advanced and inflammatory breast cancer and its link to DCE-MRI and overall survival. Int J Hyperthermia 2015;31(4): 386–95.

61. Santa-Maria CA, Camp M, Cimino-Mathews A, et al. Neoadjuvant therapy for early-stage breast cancer: current practice, controversies, and future directions. Oncology (Williston Park) 2015;29(11):828–38.

62. Mauri D, Pavlidis N, Ioannidis JP. Neoadjuvant versus adjuvant systemic treatment in breast cancer: a meta-analysis. J Natl Cancer Inst 2005; 97(3):188–94.

Problem-Solving MR Imaging for Equivocal Imaging Findings and Indeterminate Clinical Symptoms of the Breast

Ethan Cohen, MD*, Jessica W.T. Leung, MD

KEYWORDS

- Breast MR imaging • Breast cancer • MR imaging • Problem-solving MR imaging

KEY POINTS

- Problem-solving breast MR imaging strongly depends on high-quality technique and appropriate case selection.
- American and European guidelines endorse problem-solving breast MR imaging for suspicious clinical symptoms and equivocal imaging findings with limited biopsy options.
- The literature is most supportive of problem-solving breast MR imaging for pathologic nipple discharge and mammographic architectural distortion when biopsy options are limited.
- More data for breast MR imaging of calcifications, mammographic asymmetries, and surgical scarring are necessary; MR imaging has limited utility for palpable lumps, breast pain, and masses on imaging.

INTRODUCTION

Multiple imaging modalities have been developed for breast cancer screening and diagnosis. Mammography and sonography are the most widely available, and their roles in the evaluation of breast disease are relatively well defined and accepted. The role for MR imaging of the breast, however, remains somewhat controversial. The American College of Radiology's (ACR's) most recent list of indications for breast MR imaging was published in 2013[1] and included an additional evaluation for suspicion of breast cancer recurrence with inconclusive imaging as well as concerning symptoms or inconclusive imaging when biopsy cannot be performed. The ACR also clearly states that MR imaging cannot replace mammography and sonography (that is, conventional imaging) in the initial evaluation of clinical symptoms and screening mammography findings.[2] In 2015, the European Society of Breast Imaging published a similar list of MR imaging indications that also included "problem solving (equivocal findings at mammography/ultrasound) when needle biopsy cannot be performed."[3] However, MR imaging is not a routine alternative to percutaneous biopsy for suspicious imaging or suspicious clinical findings.[2,4]

There are a few obstacles to the widespread use of problem-solving breast MR imaging. The first is the high cost of the examination and the downstream evaluation of indeterminate findings.

Disclosure Statement: The authors have nothing to disclose.
Department of Diagnostic Radiology, Division of Diagnostic Imaging, The University of Texas MD Anderson Cancer Center, 1515 Holcombe Boulevard, Unit 1350, Houston, TX 77030-4009, USA
* Corresponding author.
E-mail address: ecohen@mdanderson.org

Magn Reson Imaging Clin N Am 26 (2018) 221–233
https://doi.org/10.1016/j.mric.2017.12.012
1064-9689/18/© 2017 Elsevier Inc. All rights reserved.

Although cost-benefit analyses for indications, such as high-risk screening with MR imaging, have shown a benefit,[5] data documenting long-term savings for problem-solving MR imaging are sparse.[6] Other disadvantages of MR imaging include patient anxiety, false positives, and potential morbidity from biopsy and intravenous injection of gadolinium-based contrast.

Importantly, the sensitivity, specificity, and negative predictive value (NPV) of MR imaging must be sufficiently high to maximize true positives and avoid false negatives.[7] Multiple studies show variable results for breast MR imaging performance on these measures. Three separate meta-analyses from 2008 report sensitivities of 75% to 97% and specificities of 72% to 96%.[8–10] More recent reports document sensitivities of 93% to 100% and specificities of 37% to 97%.[11] Of note, MR imaging has been found to be more sensitive for invasive carcinoma than ductal carcinoma in situ (DCIS).[12] A very high NPV is particularly important for problem-solving breast MR imaging. It is well known that MR imaging has a higher NPV than either mammography or sonography,[13] and multiple studies have reported NPVs for breast MR imaging of 91.7% to 100%.[13–17]

In particular, 2 recent reports have shown that perfect NPVs can be achieved for problem-solving breast MR imaging performed with optimal technique. In 2014, Oztekin and colleagues[18] reviewed 858 breast MR imaging examinations performed for "suspicious lesions identified by other imaging modalities or suspicious clinical findings (eg, nipple discharge or palpable abnormality)."[18] They not only found an NPV of 100% but also calculated very good sensitivity, specificity, and positive predictive value (PPV) for their series (100%, 92%, and 52%, respectively). In 2015, Spick and colleagues[19] reviewed 111 consecutive MR imaging examinations performed for inconclusive imaging findings and palpable lumps with negative imaging. They found an NPV of 100% and a PPV of 58% and concluded that breast MR imaging can reliably exclude malignancy when used for problem solving. Both studies suggest a promising role for MR imaging in these instances.

To articulate the current understanding of the utility of MR imaging for assessing suspicious symptoms and equivocal imaging findings, the authors review the current literature and guidelines regarding the use of breast MR imaging for these indications.

CLINICAL SYMPTOMS

Concerning clinical symptoms are frequent indications for breast imaging. The most common include palpable lumps, breast pain, and nipple discharge. Problem-solving MR imaging may be performed for any of these 3 symptoms, but the supporting literature is limited except for nipple discharge.

Palpable Lump

The symptom of a palpable lump most commonly represents normal dense fibroglandular breast tissue. However, a lump is also the most common presentation for symptomatic breast malignancy. The recommended initial imaging for a palpable lump includes diagnostic mammography with or without digital breast tomosynthesis (DBT) and possible sonography.[20–26] This imaging combination has shown a nearly perfect NPV of 97% to 100%.[25,27–32] Many investigators have stressed that biopsy is indicated for suspicious clinical findings despite negative conventional imaging owing to an extremely small but real risk of malignancy.[33]

However, MR imaging has limited utility for assessing lumps because it reportedly adds an unnecessary, costly step that may reduce rates of compliance with recommended follow-up.[2,33,34] Moreover, the ACR's appropriateness criteria for palpable breast masses state that the use of MR imaging during the initial evaluation is "usually not appropriate."[35]

Breast Pain (Mastodynia)

Breast pain, or mastodynia, is the most common clinical symptom seen in breast health care. Half of mastodynia cases resolve spontaneously,[36] but imaging may be necessary to exclude an underlying lesion.[37] Invasive lobular carcinoma and anaplastic carcinoma are disproportionately associated with mastodynia compared with other breast cancers,[38,39] and adenoid cystic carcinoma of the breast has been reported to present with noncyclical pain.[40]

However, mastodynia usually is not associated with breast cancer. In 1998, Dujim and colleagues[41] found no difference in the incidences of malignancy between painful breasts (0.5%), contralateral asymptomatic breasts (0.5%), and breasts of asymptomatic women referred for screening (0.7%). In 2002, Leung and colleagues[42] performed targeted sonography focusing on the site of breast pain in 110 patients in the absence of associated palpable lump and found no breast cancers, whereas Tumyan and colleagues[43] performed mammography and sonography in 86 patients with focal breast pain and no lump and found only 4 breast cancers. Two of those cancers were at the site of the tenderness (2.3%) and were visible mammographically and sonographically, whereas the other two were distant from the area of pain and presented as calcifications. The NPV of combined mammography and ultrasound for carcinoma at the site of focal pain was 100%.

Annual screening mammography is recommended by the ACR for cyclical or nonfocal breast pain, whereas diagnostic mammography with or without DBT and sonography may be appropriate in certain instances for noncyclical, unilateral, or focal breast pain.[44] The ACR clarifies that though "imaging is not routinely indicated due to the rarity of underlying cancer in this clinical scenario, it may be used in some settings to provide reassurance and to exclude a treatable benign cause for pain."[44] The ACR also notes that there are no data to suggest that breast MR imaging meets the risk-benefit or cost-effectiveness criteria for the evaluation of breast pain. Therefore, MR imaging is not recommended for mastodynia in the absence of other concerning imaging findings or clinical symptoms.

Nipple Discharge

Nipple discharge can be classified as physiologic or pathologic, and pathologic nipple discharge has the best documented role in indicating MR imaging among the symptoms reviewed in this article. Physiologic nipple discharge is bilateral, nonspontaneous, from multiple duct orifices, and white, green, or yellow. This discharge is not due to breast malignancy, and imaging is unnecessary as long as the patients' screening mammography is up to date.[45–47]

Pathologic nipple discharge is unilateral, from a single duct orifice, and serous or bloody (red or dark brown depending on chronicity). The most common cause is a papilloma (35%–48% of cases), whereas 17% to 36% of cases result from duct ectasia.[48] Malignancy is found in 5% to 21% of women with pathologic nipple discharge who undergo biopsy.[48–50]

Surgical excision of a single duct (microdochectomy) or major duct excision (removal of all the lactiferous ducts under the nipple) has historically been the treatment of choice for pathologic nipple discharge. Preoperative imaging may be helpful because up to 20% of lesions causing pathologic nipple discharge are greater than 3 cm from the nipple and may not be surgically removed. Moreover, such surgical intervention is often undesirable for women of child-bearing age.[51] The recommended initial evaluation includes diagnostic mammography with or without DBT and sonography.[45,52] The ACR confirms that breast MR imaging is "usually not appropriate"[47] in the *initial* evaluation of pathologic nipple discharge. Historically, ductography has been a helpful adjunct to conventional imaging because it detects underlying findings in 14% to 86% of cases,[52–54] even though it can be uncomfortable for patients and unsuccessful up to 10% of the time.[55] Ductography's reported sensitivity, specificity, PPV, and NPV for breast malignancy are 75% to 100%, 6% to 49%, 16% to 18%, and 93% to 100%, respectively.[51,56]

MR imaging after negative conventional imaging for pathologic nipple discharge has been extensively evaluated (**Fig. 1**). Its sensitivity for invasive breast cancer in this scenario is 86% to 100%,

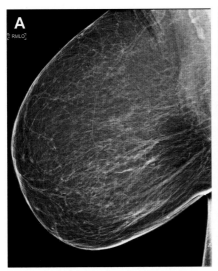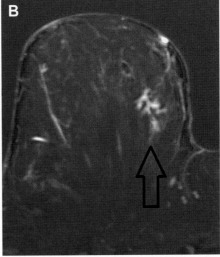

Fig. 1. A 56-year-old woman presented with spontaneous, bloody right nipple discharge. Diagnostic mammography (right mediolateral oblique view) (*A*) and sonography (not shown) were negative for malignancy. MR imaging (*B*) revealed suspicious segmental nonmass enhancement (*arrow*) in the medial right breast. MR imaging–guided biopsy yielded invasive and intraductal malignancy.

whereas its sensitivity for DCIS in this scenario is 40% to 100%.[49,53,57–60] Moreover, MR imaging identifies an underlying cause for pathologic nipple discharge in 19% to 96% of cases[53,54] and reveals suspicious posterior lesions occult to ductography. Many radiologists prefer MR imaging to ductography because of its higher NPV and PPV for carcinoma and high-risk lesions.[48,54,57,58]

Bahl and colleagues[60] recently published one of the largest studies to date of MR imaging for nipple discharge, reviewing the results for 103 women who underwent MR imaging for nipple discharge between 2004 and 2013. The sensitivity, specificity, PPV, and NPV of MR imaging in their series were 100%, 68%, 37%, and 100%, respectively; the investigators concluded that a negative MR imaging might obviate surgery given the perfect NPV.

Less supportive evidence for the use of MR imaging when nipple discharge is present has also been reported. In 2015, van Gelder and colleagues[59] reported results for 111 MR imaging examinations performed for unilateral bloody nipple discharge and found underlying breast cancer in less than 2% of patients. They concluded that MR imaging has limited value given this low rate of malignancy. Another known drawback of MR imaging for pathologic nipple discharge is that reliably differentiating carcinoma from benign processes, such as papillomas, is not possible.[61]

EQUIVOCAL IMAGING FINDINGS

Standard evaluation of screening mammography findings includes diagnostic mammography with or without DBT and may include sonography. Most findings are ultimately assessed as benign by a typically benign imaging appearance, stability over time, or percutaneous biopsy. However, some findings, including summation artifact, can be equivocal for breast malignancy; biopsy can sometimes be challenging (eg, one-view mammographic finding with no sonographic correlate). Breast MR imaging has been suggested in the literature for these instances after appropriate conventional imaging.[7,15,62] The ACR also suggests MR imaging for these scenarios and notes that MR imaging should not replace conventional imaging for screening mammography findings.[1,2] The ACR Breast Imaging Reporting and Data System (BI-RADS) Atlas restates this recommendation by stressing that "breast MR imaging is not an appropriate follow-up measure for minimal or equivocal findings."[63] Also, assessing conventional imaging as BI-RADS category 0 (incomplete: needs additional imaging assessment) is discouraged when one is recommending MR imaging for

follow-up. Instead, an assessment of BI-RADS 3 probably benign, BI-RADS 4 suspicious, or BI-RADS 5 highly suggestive of malignancy is recommended to provide an actionable assessment if the MR imaging examination is not performed.

The current recommendations from the European Society of Breast Cancer Specialists also discourage problem-solving MR imaging if percutaneous biopsy is available.[64] Similarly, the European Society of Breast Imaging's guidelines list equivocal imaging findings as a breast MR imaging indication only "when needle biopsy cannot be performed."[3] Overall, problem-solving MR imaging is best reserved for equivocal imaging findings as described later with limited options for biopsy.[65]

There are 4 types of mammographic findings in the breast, mass, calcifications, architectural distortion, and asymmetry, with varying indications for MR imaging. Careful case selection for problem-solving MR imaging is necessary to obtain high sensitivities and specificities. Historically, breast MR imaging has not been recommended for masses and calcifications, but new literature is reviewed later.

Mass

A breast mass is defined mammographically by the ACR BI-RADS Atlas as a 3-dimensional structure visible on 2 projections that has convex-outward borders and is denser at its center than near its edges.[63] Most masses are well seen with ultrasound, and histologic diagnosis is typically easily achieved with an ultrasound-guided or stereotactic biopsy (**Fig. 2**). The literature addressing MR imaging for equivocal masses is limited given the typical ease of diagnosis with conventional imaging and biopsy.

In 2014, Sarica and Uluc[4] reported findings from problem-solving MR imaging examinations performed for 277 lesions biopsied with ultrasound guidance. The NPV and PPV for MR imaging in their series were 90.7% and 68.1%, respectively. Eight breast MR imaging examinations yielded false-negative results, and the investigators concluded that MR imaging cannot obviate biopsy in cases of suspicious lesions identified by conventional imaging.

Calcifications

Calcifications are commonly identified by mammography and usually represent a benign process, such as fibrocystic change. Malignant calcifications are less common and typically represent intraductal rather than invasive malignancy.[66] The preferred imaging modality for calcifications is

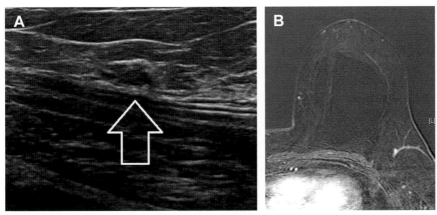

Fig. 2. A 39-year-old woman was found to have a suspicious hypoechoic mass (*arrow*) seen only sonographically (*A*) along the medial margin of her left breast implant. Biopsy was deferred owing to the proximity of the mass to the implant, and problem-solving breast MR imaging (*B*) revealed no correlate. The mass was ultimately assessed as benign after 2 years of imaging stability.

diagnostic mammography with magnification views to characterize the morphology and distribution of the calcifications. Breast MR imaging is inherently limited for assessing calcifications because it displays enhancement rather than the calcifications themselves (**Fig. 3**). Also, the sensitivity of MR imaging is lower for DCIS than for invasive cancer, especially low-grade DCIS,[12] although it has been suggested that MR imaging may help determine the extent of disease in high-grade DCIS.[61]

Early studies investigating problem-solving MR imaging for calcifications were not promising. Bazzocchi and colleagues[67] reported results in 2006 from a multicenter trial involving 112 cases of suspicious calcifications imaged with MR imaging. They found a sensitivity of 87% and an NPV of 71%, which they argued preclude routine use of MR imaging for calcifications. In 2007, Cilotti and colleagues[68] reviewed results from 55 MR imaging examinations performed for calcifications assessed as BI-RADS category 3, 4, or 5 from a single institution. With histology as the reference standard, they found an unsatisfactory NPV of 76%, though they did note that MR imaging more successfully characterized higher-grade DCIS.

In 2014, Kikuchi and colleagues[69] reviewed results from 168 consecutive patients with calcifications who underwent MR imaging before biopsy.

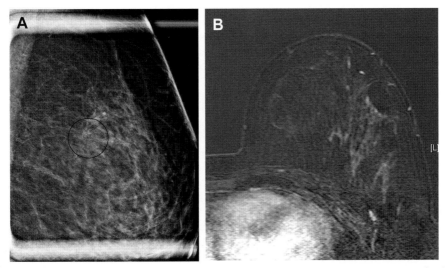

Fig. 3. A lateral magnification view (*A*) in a 42-year-old woman revealed a suspicious group of calcifications (*circle*) in the upper outer left breast. Problem-solving MR imaging (*B*) performed before biopsy at the referring physician's request was negative, and stereotactic biopsy revealed fibrocystic changes.

The sensitivity, specificity, PPV, and NPV for MR imaging in their series were 84%, 82%, 58%, and 95%, respectively; they concluded that the NPV was sufficiently high to consider MR imaging for triaging cases before biopsy. Data from a systematic review and meta-analysis published in 2017 also suggest MR imaging may be useful for assessing calcifications.[70] Twenty studies meeting the inclusion criteria yielded 1843 cases of calcifications assessed as BI-RADS category 3, 4, or 5 that were evaluated with MR imaging (40.6% malignant). The calculated sensitivity and specificity of MR imaging for all calcifications (BI-RADS category 3, 4, and 5) were 87% and 81%, respectively; yet, the calculated sensitivity and specificity of MR imaging for BI-RADS category 4 calcifications were 92% and 82%, respectively. Using enhancement as the diagnostic criteria, the investigators recommended against using breast MR imaging for BI-RADS category 3 or 5 calcifications but stated that breast MR imaging may be considered for category 4 calcifications.

Further study of BI-RADS category 4 calcifications was also reported in 2017. Bennani-Baiti and colleagues[71] reviewed 248 consecutive breast MR imaging examinations performed for BI-RADS category 4 calcifications identified at mammography. The calculated PPV and NPV were excellent (80.5% and 96.7%, respectively), and only 4 false negative examinations were encountered (3 BI-RADS category 4c calcifications and one BI-RADS category 4b calcifications). These observations led to the conclusion that MR imaging may be used to identify cases of BI-RADS category 4a and 4b calcifications in which biopsy may be obviated.

A retrospective study ahead of print at time of this writing also concluded that MR imaging might help reduce unnecessary biopsies for calcifications and that MR imaging may be able to distinguish between malignant and benign calcifications.[72] Baltzer and colleagues[72] reviewed data from 152 patients with suspicious calcifications on mammography who underwent problem-solving MR imaging before biopsy. They reported sensitivity, specificity, and NPV for MR imaging in this setting of 97.2%, 39.5%, and 94.1%, respectively.

Overall, though problem-solving breast MR imaging is not routinely recommended for calcifications at this time, further investigation may be warranted as techniques and costs improve. A role for breast MR imaging in diagnosing breast calcifications may evolve as more data come forth.

Architectural Distortion

Architectural distortion is defined mammographically by the ACR BI-RADS Atlas as distorted tissue with "thin straight lines or spiculations radiating from a focal point, and focal retraction, distortion, or straightening at the anterior or posterior edge of the parenchyma."[63] The most common cause is prior surgery or trauma, but malignancy can produce a desmoplastic reaction and distort adjacent parenchyma mammographically. Architectural distortion is estimated to account for 6% of abnormalities at screening and is the third most common imaging appearance of malignancy at mammography.[73,74] Other benign causes of architectural distortion include radial scar/complex sclerosing lesion, fibrosis, sclerosing adenosis, and, rarely, granular cell tumor.[73,75] Architectural distortion without an apparent benign cause always requires further workup.

A complete understanding of the causes and appropriate workup of architectural distortion is particularly important in the era of DBT. Previously mammographically occult distortions are frequently identified with DBT. In 2014, Partyka and colleagues[76] reported the results of 9982 screening mammograms performed with DBT and noted that 73% of the identified architectural distortions were seen on only the DBT portion of the examination. They and other investigators have found that architectural distortion without a sonographic correlate is more likely to represent a radial scar than malignancy.[77]

MR imaging has been studied as a problem-solving tool for mammographic architectural distortion. In 2009, Perfetto and colleagues[78] reported results from MR imaging examinations performed for architectural distortion in 20 patients. The calculated NPV of 100% led them to conclude that breast MR imaging may identify cases of radial scars that do not need to be surgically excised. More recently, in 2016, Si and colleagues[75] reviewed the diagnostic accuracy of dynamic contrast-enhanced breast MR imaging and apparent diffusion coefficient values for 57 cases of mammographic architectural distortion and found a sensitivity of 92.9% and a specificity of 79.3% for the combination of dynamic contrast-enhanced breast MR imaging and apparent diffusion coefficient values using 0.61 as the threshold for the normalized apparent diffusion coefficient. They concluded that this imaging combination was more reliable than mammography.

Management of architectural distortion on one mammographic projection only and/or without an ultrasound correlate can be challenging. MR imaging may play a role here, though data remain sparse (**Fig. 4**). In 2016, Durand and colleagues[79] proposed a workup algorithm: Percutaneous biopsy after complete evaluation with mammography/DBT and sonography is recommended.

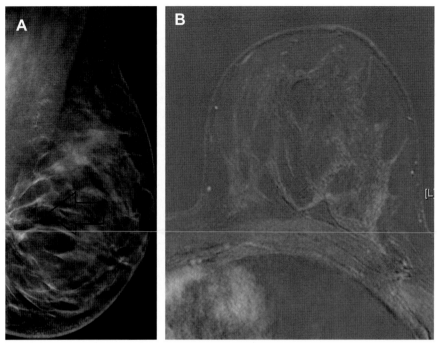

Fig. 4. A 33-year-old woman was found to have sonographically occult, one-view-only architectural distortion (*arrow*) on the DBT portion only (left mediolateral oblique view) (*A*) of her baseline mammogram. The location was deemed not amenable to DBT-guided biopsy, and problem-solving breast MR imaging (*B*) was negative for evidence of breast malignancy. The distortion remained mammographically stable for more than 2 years.

Ultrasound guidance for biopsy is preferred, but stereotactic biopsy can be considered if the architectural distortion is clearly seen on standard mammographic views. A DBT-guided biopsy is indicated for architectural distortion seen only on DBT, and an MR imaging possibly followed by MR imaging–guided biopsy can be performed if DBT-guided biopsy is unavailable. Short-term follow-up imaging and excisional biopsy following DBT-guided localization are other options at the radiologist's discretion.

It should be noted that there are no robust, evidence-based guidelines for managing questionable or subtle architectural distortion with no MR imaging or ultrasound correlate. Further studies are needed to clarify the role of MR imaging and short-term follow-up imaging for architectural distortion, especially when the distortion is identified only on DBT and/or on only one mammographic projection.

Asymmetry

Four types of mammographic asymmetries exist in the current version of BI-RADS.[63] The first is an asymmetry, defined as prominent fibroglandular-density tissue on only one mammographic projection and typically represents summation.

Asymmetric fibroglandular-density tissue occupying at least one quadrant of the breast is referred to as a global asymmetry, typically a normal variant. A focal asymmetry is a small amount of fibroglandular-density tissue that has a similar shape on at least 2 mammographic projections, lacks the convex-outward borders and conspicuity of a mass, and often contains interspersed fat. The final and most suspicious type of asymmetry is a developing asymmetry, which is defined as a new or enlarging focal asymmetry.[80]

The following likelihoods of malignancy for each type were reported in 2007: asymmetry, 1.8%; nonpalpable global asymmetry, 0%; palpable global asymmetry, 7.5%; focal asymmetry, 0.67%; and developing asymmetry, 12.8%.[81] In 2009, Venkatesan and colleagues[82] described slightly higher PPVs for asymmetries and focal asymmetries from screening (3.6% and 3.7%, respectively) and noted that developing asymmetries were more likely to represent malignancy at diagnostic mammography (PPV: 19.7%) than at screening mammography (PPV: 7.4%).

Data supporting problem-solving MR imaging examinations performed for asymmetries are limited. One of the largest studies to date that involved this role for MR imaging focused on developing asymmetries[83]: in 2016, Chesebro and colleagues[83] reviewed 2354 consecutive diagnostic mammograms and identified 202 developing asymmetries. Thirty-one were malignant (15.3%), and MR imaging was performed for 66 of the 202 lesions. All malignant developing asymmetries imaged with MR imaging (10 of 10) had an MR imaging correlate, whereas only 15 of 53 benign developing asymmetries imaged with MR imaging had an MR imaging correlate ($P<.0001$). The investigators concluded that an MR imaging correlate was predictive of malignancy. However, further studies are needed to clarify the role of problem-solving MR imaging for all types of asymmetries.

Empirical data

There are reasonable data for problem-solving MR imaging of equivocal imaging findings. However, further studies are needed to produce results that can affect clinical practice.

Early work by Orel and colleagues[84] in 1996 suggested that MR imaging may be useful for one-view-only mammographic findings and equivocal changes at prior biopsy sites. Sardanelli and colleagues[85] evaluated 19 patients with inconclusive imaging findings who underwent MR imaging in the 1990s. The evaluation showed 5 malignancies and resulted in one false negative and 2 false positives, which led the investigators to suggest that MR imaging is a useful problem-solving tool. A larger study in 1999 by Lee and colleagues[86] reported 86 MR imaging examinations performed for equivocal mammographic findings. Two-thirds of the findings were asymmetries, and one-third were architectural distortions. Twenty-six MR imaging examinations revealed a correlate for the equivocal findings; 12 incidental lesions were encountered; and 10 breast malignancies were diagnosed from positive MR imaging examinations. The mammographic findings without an MR imaging correlate were benign at excision or mammographically stable (mean: 19 months), and the investigators concluded that adjunctive MR imaging has value for problematic mammographic findings.

A prospective, multicenter trial of the International Breast MR Consortium performed from June 1998 through October 2001 involved 821 patients with suspicious imaging or clinical findings who underwent MR imaging before biopsy.[87] Four hundred four malignancies (63 DCISs and 341 invasive carcinomas) were diagnosed; the sensitivity, specificity, and area under the receiver operator characteristic curve for MR imaging were 88.1%, 67.7%, and 0.88, respectively. The calculated PPV for MR imaging was higher than that of mammography (72.4% vs 52.8%; $P<.005$), and the NPV for MR imaging was 85.4%. The

investigators concluded that this NPV was too low to forgo biopsy in cases of suspicious imaging and clinical findings.

In 2009, Moy and colleagues[15] reported results for 115 MR imaging examinations performed for inconclusive imaging findings not amenable to percutaneous biopsy. One hundred MR imaging examinations revealed no correlate for the index finding, whereas 6 of the remaining 15 MR imaging examinations revealed a malignant correlate for the index finding. The investigators found a higher specificity, PPV, and accuracy for MR imaging than for mammography and concluded that MR imaging is useful for appropriately selected equivocal imaging findings.

Dorrius and colleagues[88] reviewed the literature for MR imaging of probably benign calcified and noncalcified mammographic findings in 2010. Of the 5 studies included, 2 reported an NPV of 100% for MR imaging of noncalcified BI-RADS category 3 findings. The remaining 3, which focused exclusively on MR imaging of probably benign calcifications, revealed an NPV of 76% to 97%; the investigators concluded that adjunctive MR imaging is reliable for noncalcified BI-RADS category 3 mammographic findings.

In 2015, Spick and colleagues[19] reported results from 111 MR imaging examinations performed for 109 inconclusive imaging findings and 2 palpable lumps without imaging correlates. Their reference standard was histopathology or 1 year of imaging stability, and 15 breast malignancies were diagnosed. The sensitivity, specificity, and NPV for MR imaging in their cohort were 100%, 88.5%, and 100%, respectively; the investigators concluded that MR imaging reliably excludes malignancy in patients with equivocal imaging and clinical findings.

Finally, a systematic review and meta-analysis from 2016 also found an NPV of 100% for MR imaging performed for noncalcified imaging findings using the same reference standard as Spick and colleagues.[89] Included were 2316 lesions from 14 studies, and the investigators also concluded that MR imaging may be useful for equivocal, noncalcified imaging findings.

The data on the utility of problem-solving MR imaging for equivocal conventional imaging of the breast are clearly heterogeneous. Further studies are indicated to determine the cost-effectiveness and utility of problem-solving MR imaging for this purpose, as most available data are from retrospective studies with inherent limited generalizability.

Surgical scar

Differentiating malignancy from surgical scarring, especially at the location of treated breast cancer, can be challenging because carcinoma can appear mammographically and sonographically identical to surgical changes.[90] In fact, diagnosing recurrent breast cancer can be more difficult than identifying the original tumor because of the presence of scar tissue[91]; the sensitivity of mammography for recurrence in the treated breast is 55% to 68%.[90]

The ACR includes suspected breast cancer recurrence as an indication for MR imaging and reports that it may be useful "when clinical, mammographic, and/or sonographic findings are inconclusive."[1] However, neither the National Comprehensive Cancer Network nor the American Society of Clinical Oncology recommend routine use of MR imaging after breast conservation surgery.[92]

Early literature from the 1990s suggested that MR imaging helps distinguish scarring from malignancy.[93–95] Two series from 2002 and 2006 with less than 100 postoperative patients reported sensitivities of 90% to 100% and NPVs of 98.7% to 100% for MR imaging.[96,97] In 2010, Rinaldi and colleagues[98] described results from MR imaging with diffusion-weighted imaging in 72 patients with suspected recurrence at their lumpectomy site. The investigators found that the mean apparent diffusion coefficient value for recurrence was lower than for scarring ($P<.001$) and concluded that diffusion-weighted imaging may help differentiate between scarring and malignancy. However, there was no pathologic evaluation when the MR imaging was negative, and the mean longitudinal follow-up was only 6 months. Further studies are warranted to confirm these findings.

Examination timing is very important when one is evaluating for local recurrence. Evidence suggests that MR imaging performed at least 12 to 18 months after surgery is optimal and yields a sensitivity of 90% to 100% and specificity of 83% to 93%.[90] No enhancement at the surgical site suggests benign fibrosis, whereas enhancement at the surgical site warrants further evaluation, particularly if the surgery took place more than 1 year ago. But even with optimal timing, minimal normal focal enhancement or thin linear nonmass enhancement can persist at the surgical site for up to 18 months or, rarely, beyond 5 years.[99]

LIMITATIONS

Breast MR imaging is a powerful imaging tool because of its high sensitivity and NPV when performed with optimal technique. However, it is typically less specific because benign processes can appear similar to malignancy. Incidental false positives are common, increase costs, and cause undue patient anxiety and morbidity. These ramifications are magnified with problem-solving MR imaging because of the lower probability of malignancy compared with other indications. Prudent case selection is essential.

Other limitations include the subjectivity of MR imaging interpretation and challenges correlating MR imaging findings with conventional imaging. A thorough review of the patients' recent breast imaging is paramount for accurate problem-solving MR imaging. Finally, MR imaging can be fraught with technical issues that can limit the diagnostic quality of the images.[100] Prioritizing high image quality will enable high diagnostic performance.

SUMMARY

The ACR and other organizations endorse problem-solving MR imaging for certain clinical and equivocal imaging findings, especially when biopsy options are limited. Appropriate case selection is crucial, and MR imaging should be performed only after appropriate evaluation with conventional imaging. Overall, MR imaging is best reserved for cases of pathologic nipple discharge and sonographically occult architectural distortion with limited biopsy options. Further study is necessary to define the role of problem-solving MR imaging for calcifications, mammographic asymmetries, and surgical scarring; minimal to no utility is likely for palpable lumps, breast pain, and masses on imaging.

REFERENCES

1. ACR practice parameter for the performance of contrast-enhanced magnetic resonance imaging (MRI) of the breast. Available at: https://www.acr.org/~/media/2a0eb28eb59041e2825179afb72ef624.pdf. Accessed February 8, 2017.
2. Yau EJ, Gutierrez RL, DeMartini WB, et al. The utility of breast MRI as a problem-solving tool. Breast J 2011;17(3):273–80.
3. Mann RM, Balleyguier C, Baltzer PA, et al. Breast MRI: EUSOBI recommendations for women's information. Eur Radiol 2015;25(12):3669–78.
4. Sarica O, Uluc F. Additional diagnostic value of MRI in patients with suspicious breast lesions based on ultrasound. Br J Radiol 2014;87(1041): 20140009.
5. Griebsch I, Brown J, Boggis C, et al. Cost-effectiveness of screening with contrast enhanced magnetic resonance imaging vs X-ray mammography of women at a high familial risk of breast cancer. Br J Cancer 2006;95(7):801–10.

6. DeMartini W, Lehman C. A review of current evidence-based clinical applications for breast magnetic resonance imaging. Top Magn Reson Imaging 2008;19(3):143–50.

7. Leung JW. MR imaging in the evaluation of equivocal clinical and imaging findings of the breast. Magn Reson Imaging Clin N Am 2010;18(2):295–308, ix–x.

8. Peters NH, Borel Rinkes IH, Zuithoff NP, et al. Meta-analysis of MR imaging in the diagnosis of breast lesions. Radiology 2008;246(1):116–24.

9. Warner E, Messersmith H, Causer P, et al. Systematic review: using magnetic resonance imaging to screen women at high risk for breast cancer. Ann Intern Med 2008;148(9):671–9.

10. Granader EJ, Dwamena B, Carlos RC. MRI and mammography surveillance of women at increased risk for breast cancer: recommendations using an evidence-based approach. Acad Radiol 2008;15(12):1590–5.

11. Comstock C, Sung J. CAD for breast MRI. In: Molleran V, Mahoney M, editors. Breast MRI. Philadelphia: Elsevier Saunders; 2014. p. 24–31.

12. Morrow M, Waters J, Morris E. MRI for breast cancer screening, diagnosis, and treatment. Lancet 2011;378(9805):1804–11.

13. Vassiou K, Kanavou T, Vlychou M, et al. Characterization of breast lesions with CE-MR multimodal morphological and kinetic analysis: comparison with conventional mammography and high-resolution ultrasound. Eur J Radiol 2009;70(1):69–76.

14. Gokalp G, Topal U. MR imaging in probably benign lesions (BI-RADS category 3) of the breast. Eur J Radiol 2006;57(3):436–44.

15. Moy L, Elias K, Patel V, et al. Is breast MRI helpful in the evaluation of inconclusive mammographic findings? AJR Am J Roentgenol 2009;193(4):986–93.

16. Kuhl CK, Schmutzler RK, Leutner CC, et al. Breast MR imaging screening in 192 women proved or suspected to be carriers of a breast cancer susceptibility gene: preliminary results. Radiology 2000;215(1):267–79.

17. Dorrius MD, Pijnappel RM, Sijens PE, et al. The negative predictive value of breast magnetic resonance imaging in noncalcified BIRADS 3 lesions. Eur J Radiol 2012;81(2):209–13.

18. Oztekin PS, Kosar PN. Magnetic resonance imaging of the breast as a problem-solving method: to be or not to be? Breast J 2014;20(6):622–31.

19. Spick C, Szolar DH, Preidler KW, et al. Breast MRI used as a problem-solving tool reliably excludes malignancy. Eur J Radiol 2015;84(1):61–4.

20. Ciatto S, Houssami N. Breast imaging and needle biopsy in women with clinically evident breast cancer: does combined imaging change overall diagnostic sensitivity? Breast 2007;16(4):382–6.

21. Murphy IG, Dillon MF, Doherty AO, et al. Analysis of patients with false negative mammography and symptomatic breast carcinoma. J Surg Oncol 2007;96(6):457–63.

22. Noroozian M, Hadjiiski L, Rahnama-Moghadam S, et al. Digital breast tomosynthesis is comparable to mammographic spot views for mass characterization. Radiology 2012;262(1):61–8.

23. Skaane P, Gullien R, Bjorndal H, et al. Digital breast tomosynthesis (DBT): initial experience in a clinical setting. Acta Radiol 2012;53(5):524–9.

24. Harvey JA. Sonography of palpable breast masses. Semin Ultrasound CT MR 2006;27(4):284–97.

25. Shetty MK, Shah YP, Sharman RS. Prospective evaluation of the value of combined mammographic and sonographic assessment in patients with palpable abnormalities of the breast. J Ultrasound Med 2003;22(3):263–8 [quiz: 269–70].

26. American College of Radiology (ACR) appropriateness criteria® palpable breast masses. Available at: https://acsearch.acr.org/docs/69495/Narrative/. Accessed February 9, 2017.

27. Soo MS, Rosen EL, Baker JA, et al. Negative predictive value of sonography with mammography in patients with palpable breast lesions. AJR Am J Roentgenol 2001;177(5):1167–70.

28. Moy L, Slanetz PJ, Moore R, et al. Specificity of mammography and US in the evaluation of a palpable abnormality: retrospective review. Radiology 2002;225(1):176–81.

29. Moss HA, Britton PD, Flower CD, et al. How reliable is modern breast imaging in differentiating benign from malignant breast lesions in the symptomatic population? Clin Radiol 1999;54(10):676–82.

30. Gumus H, Gumus M, Mills P, et al. Clinically palpable breast abnormalities with normal imaging: is clinically guided biopsy still required? Clin Radiol 2012;67(5):437–40.

31. Dennis MA, Parker SH, Klaus AJ, et al. Breast biopsy avoidance: the value of normal mammograms and normal sonograms in the setting of a palpable lump. Radiology 2001;219(1):186–91.

32. Lehman CD, Lee CI, Loving VA, et al. Accuracy and value of breast ultrasound for primary imaging evaluation of symptomatic women 30-39 years of age. AJR Am J Roentgenol 2012;199(5):1169–77.

33. Lehman CD, Lee AY, Lee CI. Imaging management of palpable breast abnormalities. AJR Am J Roentgenol 2014;203(5):1142–53.

34. Olsen ML, Morton MJ, Stan DL, et al. Is there a role for magnetic resonance imaging in diagnosing palpable breast masses when mammogram and ultrasound are negative? J Womens Health (Larchmt) 2012;21(11):1149–54.

35. American College of Radiology ACR appropriateness criteria® palpable breast masses. Available at: https://acsearch.acr.org/docs/69495/Narrative/. Accessed February 8, 2017.

36. Maddox PR, Harrison BJ, Mansel RE, et al. Non-cyclical mastalgia: an improved classification and treatment. Br J Surg 1989;76(9):901–4.

37. Davies EL, Gateley CA, Miers M, et al. The long-term course of mastalgia. J R Soc Med 1998; 91(9):462–4.

38. Preece PE, Baum M, Mansel RE, et al. Importance of mastalgia in operable breast cancer. Br Med J (Clin Res Ed) 1982;284(6325):1299–300.

39. Chiedozie LC, Guirguis MN. Mastalgia and breast tumour in Nigerian women. West Afr J Med 1990; 9(1):54–8.

40. McClenathan JH, de la Roza G. Adenoid cystic breast cancer. Am J Surg 2002;183(6):646–9.

41. Duijm LE, Guit GL, Hendriks JH, et al. Value of breast imaging in women with painful breasts: observational follow up study. BMJ 1998; 317(7171):1492–5.

42. Leung JW, Kornguth PJ, Gotway MB. Utility of targeted sonography in the evaluation of focal breast pain. J Ultrasound Med 2002;21(5):521–6 [quiz: 528–9].

43. Tumyan L, Hoyt AC, Bassett LW. Negative predictive value of sonography and mammography in patients with focal breast pain. Breast J 2005;11(5): 333–7.

44. American College of Radiology ACR appropriateness criteria® breast pain. Available at: https:// acsearch.acr.org/docs/3091546/Narrative/. Accessed February 9, 2017.

45. Gray RJ, Pockaj BA, Karstaedt PJ. Navigating murky waters: a modern treatment algorithm for nipple discharge. Am J Surg 2007;194(6):850–4 [discussion: 854–5].

46. Gulay H, Bora S, Kilicturgay S, et al. Management of nipple discharge. J Am Coll Surg 1994;178(5): 471–4.

47. American College of Radiology ACR appropriateness criteria® evaluation of nipple discharge. Available at: https://acsearch.acr.org/docs/3099312/ Narrative/. Accessed February 13, 2017.

48. Orel SG, Dougherty CS, Reynolds C, et al. MR imaging in patients with nipple discharge: initial experience. Radiology 2000;216(1):248–54.

49. Lorenzon M, Zuiani C, Linda A, et al. Magnetic resonance imaging in patients with nipple discharge: should we recommend it? Eur Radiol 2011;21(5):899–907.

50. Bahl M, Baker JA, Greenup RA, et al. Diagnostic value of ultrasound in female patients with nipple discharge. AJR Am J Roentgenol 2015;205(1): 203–8.

51. Cabioglu N, Hunt KK, Singletary SE, et al. Surgical decision making and factors determining a diagnosis of breast carcinoma in women presenting with nipple discharge. J Am Coll Surg 2003; 196(3):354–64.

52. Morrogh M, Park A, Elkin EB, et al. Lessons learned from 416 cases of nipple discharge of the breast. Am J Surg 2010;200(1):73–80.

53. Morrogh M, Morris EA, Liberman L, et al. The predictive value of ductography and magnetic resonance imaging in the management of nipple discharge. Ann Surg Oncol 2007;14(12):3369–77.

54. Lubina N, Schedelbeck U, Roth A, et al. 3.0 Tesla breast magnetic resonance imaging in patients with nipple discharge when mammography and ultrasound fail. Eur Radiol 2015;25(5):1285–93.

55. Sickles EA. Galactography and other imaging investigations of nipple discharge. Lancet 2000; 356(9242):1622–3.

56. Adepoju LJ, Chun J, El-Tamer M, et al. The value of clinical characteristics and breast-imaging studies in predicting a histopathologic diagnosis of cancer or high-risk lesion in patients with spontaneous nipple discharge. Am J Surg 2005;190(4):644–6.

57. Nakahara H, Namba K, Watanabe R, et al. A comparison of MR imaging, galactography and ultrasonography in patients with nipple discharge. Breast Cancer 2003;10(4):320–9.

58. Manganaro L, D'Ambrosio I, Gigli S, et al. Breast MRI in patients with unilateral bloody and serous-bloody nipple discharge: a comparison with galactography. Biomed Res Int 2015;2015:806368.

59. van Gelder L, Bisschops RH, Menke-Pluymers MB, et al. Magnetic resonance imaging in patients with unilateral bloody nipple discharge; useful when conventional diagnostics are negative? World J Surg 2015;39(1):184–6.

60. Bahl M, Baker JA, Greenup RA, et al. Evaluation of pathologic nipple discharge: what is the added diagnostic value of MRI? Ann Surg Oncol 2015; 22(Suppl 3):S435–41.

61. Kuhl CK. Current status of breast MR imaging. Part 2. Clinical applications. Radiology 2007;244(3):672–91.

62. Lee CH. Problem solving MR imaging of the breast. Radiologic Clin 2004;42(5):919–34.

63. D'Orsi C, Sickles E, Mendelson E, et al. ACR BI-RADS ® atlas, breast imaging reporting and data system. Reston (VA): American College of Radiology; 2013.

64. Sardanelli F, Boetes C, Borisch B, et al. Magnetic resonance imaging of the breast: recommendations from the EUSOMA working group. Eur J Cancer 2010;46(8):1296–316.

65. Giess CS, Chikarmane SA, Sippo DA, et al. Breast MR imaging for equivocal mammographic findings: help or hindrance? Radiographics 2016;36(4):943–56.

66. Stomper PC, Margolin FR. Ductal carcinoma in situ: the mammographer's perspective. AJR Am J Roentgenol 1994;162(3):585–91.

67. Bazzocchi M, Zuiani C, Panizza P, et al. Contrast-enhanced breast MRI in patients with suspicious microcalcifications on mammography: results of a

multicenter trial. AJR Am J Roentgenol 2006; 186(6):1723–32.

68. Cilotti A, Iacconi C, Marini C, et al. Contrast-enhanced MR imaging in patients with BI-RADS 3-5 microcalcifications. Radiol Med 2007;112(2):272–86.

69. Kikuchi M, Tanino H, Kosaka Y, et al. Usefulness of MRI of microcalcification lesions to determine the indication for stereotactic mammotome biopsy. Anticancer Res 2014;34(11):6749–53.

70. Bennani-Baiti B, Baltzer P. MR imaging for diagnosis of malignancy in mammographic microcalcifications: a systematic review and meta-analysis. Radiology 2017;283(3):692–701.

71. Bennani-Baiti B, Dietzel M, Baltzer P. MRI for the assessment of malignancy in BI-RADS 4 mammographic microcalcifications. PLoS One 2017; 12(11):e0188679.

72. Baltzer PAT, Bennani-Baiti B, Stottinger A, et al. Is breast MRI a helpful additional diagnostic test in suspicious mammographic microcalcifications? Magn Reson Imaging 2018;46:70–4.

73. Gaur S, Dialani V, Slanetz PJ, et al. Architectural distortion of the breast. AJR Am J Roentgenol 2013;201(5):W662–70.

74. Digabel-Chabay C, Allioux C, Labbe-Devilliers C, et al. Architectural distortion and diagnostic difficulties. J Radiol 2004;85(12 Pt 2):2099–106 [in French].

75. Si L, Zhai R, Liu X, et al. MRI in the differential diagnosis of primary architectural distortion detected by mammography. Diagn Interv Radiol 2016;22(2): 141–50.

76. Partyka L, Lourenco AP, Mainiero MB. Detection of mammographically occult architectural distortion on digital breast tomosynthesis screening: initial clinical experience. AJR Am J Roentgenol 2014; 203(1):216–22.

77. Freer PE, Niell B, Rafferty EA. Preoperative tomosynthesis-guided needle localization of mammographically and sonographically occult breast lesions. Radiology 2015;275(2):377–83.

78. Perfetto F, Fiorentino F, Urbano F, et al. Adjunctive diagnostic value of MRI in the breast radial scar. Radiol Med 2009;114(5):757–70.

79. Durand MA, Wang S, Hooley RJ, et al. Tomosynthesis-detected architectural distortion: management algorithm with radiologic-pathologic correlation. Radiographics 2016;36(2):311–21.

80. Leung JW, Sickles EA. Developing asymmetry identified on mammography: correlation with imaging outcome and pathologic findings. AJR Am J Roentgenol 2007;188(3):667–75.

81. Sickles EA. The spectrum of breast asymmetries: imaging features, work-up, management. Radiol Clin North Am 2007;45(5):765–71, v.

82. Venkatesan A, Chu P, Kerlikowske K, et al. Positive predictive value of specific mammographic findings according to reader and patient variables. Radiology 2009;250(3):648–57.

83. Chesebro AL, Winkler NS, Birdwell RL, et al. Developing asymmetry at mammography: correlation with US and MR imaging and histopathologic findings. Radiology 2016;279(2):385–94.

84. Orel SG, Hochman MG, Schnall MD, et al. High-resolution MR imaging of the breast: clinical context. Radiographics 1996;16(6):1385–401.

85. Sardanelli F, Melani E, Ottonello C, et al. Magnetic resonance imaging of the breast in characterizing positive or uncertain mammographic findings. Cancer Detect Prev 1998;22(1):39–42.

86. Lee CH, Smith RC, Levine JA, et al. Clinical usefulness of MR imaging of the breast in the evaluation of the problematic mammogram. AJR Am J Roentgenol 1999;173(5):1323–9.

87. Bluemke DA, Gatsonis CA, Chen MH, et al. Magnetic resonance imaging of the breast prior to biopsy. Jama 2004;292(22):2735–42.

88. Dorrius M, Pijnappel R, Jansen-van der Weide M, et al. Breast magnetic resonance imaging as a problem-solving modality in mammographic BI-RADS 3 lesions. Cancer Imaging 2010;10(Spec no A):S54–8.

89. Bennani-Baiti B, Bennani-Baiti N, Baltzer PA. Diagnostic performance of breast magnetic resonance imaging in non-calcified equivocal breast findings: results from a systematic review and meta-analysis. PLoS One 2016;11(8):e0160346.

90. Chansakul T, Lai KC, Slanetz PJ. The postconservation breast: part 2, imaging findings of tumor recurrence and other long-term sequelae. AJR Am J Roentgenol 2012;198(2):331–43.

91. Mendelson EB. Evaluation of the postoperative breast. Radiol Clin North Am 1992;30(1):107–38.

92. Schneble EJ, Graham LJ, Shupe MP, et al. Current approaches and challenges in early detection of breast cancer recurrence. J Cancer 2014;5(4): 281–90.

93. Kerslake RW, Fox JN, Carleton PJ, et al. Dynamic contrast-enhanced and fat suppressed magnetic resonance imaging in suspected recurrent carcinoma of the breast: preliminary experience. Br J Radiol 1994;67(804):1158–68.

94. Whitehouse GH, Moore NR. MR imaging of the breast after surgery for breast cancer. Magn Reson Imaging Clin N Am 1994;2(4):591–603.

95. Muuller RD, Barkhausen J, Sauerwein W, et al. Assessment of local recurrence after breast-conserving therapy with MRI. J Comput Assist Tomogr 1998;22(3):408–12.

96. Belli P, Costantini M, Romani M, et al. Magnetic resonance imaging in breast cancer recurrence. Breast Cancer Res Treat 2002;73(3):223–35.

97. Preda L, Villa G, Rizzo S, et al. Magnetic resonance mammography in the evaluation of recurrence at

the prior lumpectomy site after conservative surgery and radiotherapy. Breast Cancer Res 2006;
8(5):R53.

98. Rinaldi P, Giuliani M, Belli P, et al. DWI in breast MRI:
role of ADC value to determine diagnosis between
recurrent tumor and surgical scar in operated patients. Eur J Radiol 2010;75(2):e114–23.

99. Drukteinis JS, Gombos EC, Raza S, et al. MR imaging assessment of the breast after breast conservation therapy: distinguishing benign from malignant
lesions. Radiographics 2012;32(1):219–34.

100. Westbrook C. Handbook of MRI technique. 4th edition. Chichester (West Sussex): John Wiley & Sons,
Ltd; 2014.

MR Imaging–Guided Breast Interventions
Indications, Key Principles, and Imaging-Pathology Correlation

Lumarie Santiago, MD*, Rosalind P. Candelaria, MD,
Monica L. Huang, MD

KEYWORDS

- Breast biopsy • Breast MR imaging • Preoperative needle localization • MR imaging guidance
- Imaging-pathology correlation

KEY POINTS

- MR imaging–guided breast interventions, including biopsy, clip placement, and preoperative needle localization, are safe, accurate, and effective.
- Mastery of the key principles of MR imaging–guided breast interventions ensure technical success with minimal patient discomfort and minimal complications.
- Imaging-pathology correlation after MR imaging–guided biopsy is essential to confirm accurate sampling and to guide creation of a multidisciplinary management plan.

INTRODUCTION

MR imaging has been used for breast cancer screening and staging since the 1990s. MR imaging has a sensitivity ranging from 86% to 100% in the detection of breast lesions, but considerable overlap in the appearance of benign and malignant lesions remains.[1,2] Therefore, tissue diagnosis of suspicious MR imaging–detected breast lesions is required. MR imaging–guided biopsy allows tissue diagnosis when suspicious MR imaging findings are mammographically and sonographically occult.[3,4] MR imaging–guided preoperative clip placement and needle localization also allow localization of suspicious MR imaging–detected lesions requiring surgical excision not amenable to MR imaging–guided biopsy.[5,6] These MR imaging–guided interventions have been proved safe, accurate, and effective.[5–11] Although fine-needle aspiration and automated core needles were previously used for biopsy, the current preferred biopsy device is a vacuum-assisted needle

owing to concerns regarding sampling adequacy and imaging-pathology concordance with the other biopsy methods.[12,13] The American College of Radiology instituted accreditation for breast MR imaging in 2010 and requires facilities that perform breast MR imaging to have equipment to perform MR imaging–guided interventions or have a referral arrangement with another facility to do so.[14,15]

This article reviews the indications for MR imaging–guided breast biopsy, clip placement, and preoperative needle localization; reviews the equipment and key steps necessary for successfully performing such interventions; and discusses the importance of postprocedure imaging-pathology correlation.

INDICATIONS FOR MR IMAGING–GUIDED BREAST INTERVENTIONS

MR imaging–guided biopsy is indicated for suspicious MR imaging–detected breast lesions, that is,

Disclosure Statement: The authors have nothing to disclose.
Department of Radiology, The University of Texas MD Anderson Cancer Center, 1515 Holcombe Boulevard, Unit 1350, Houston, TX 77030, USA
* Corresponding author.
E-mail address: lumarie.santiago@mdanderson.org

Magn Reson Imaging Clin N Am 26 (2018) 235–246
https://doi.org/10.1016/j.mric.2017.12.002

lesions assessed as Breast Imaging Reporting and Data System (BI-RADS) 4 (suspicious) or 5 (highly suggestive of malignancy) that have uncertain sonographic or mammographic correlates and lesions only or best visualized on MR imaging.[16]

It may be difficult, however, to identify a mammographic or sonographic correlate for a suspicious MR imaging–detected lesion because of the differences in patient positioning among these imaging modalities. Understanding the relationships of an MR imaging–detected lesion to the skin, pectoralis muscle, and chest wall as well as its clock position and distance from the nipple facilitates identification of a correlate by sonography or mammography.[17,18] In breasts that are predominantly fatty, the lesion displacement may be greater than expected on sonography than on MR imaging; thus, breast tissue composition also needs to be taken into account.[17,18]

If biopsy is not feasible due to lesion location or patient or referring physician preference, MR imaging–guided preoperative needle localization followed by surgical excision is an option. Alternatively, MR imaging–guided clip placement followed by mammography-guided needle or radioactive seed localization may also be performed.

PREPROCEDURE EVENTS
Procedure Planning

Before any MR imaging–guided intervention, the diagnostic breast MR imaging should be reviewed to assess the feasibility of the requested intervention, the need for intravenous contrast agent administration, and the timing of optimal lesion visualization. Biopsy may not be feasible if the lesion is close to the skin or nipple or if markedly posterior, particularly when medially located. Some lesions have an anatomic correlate on precontrast T1 imaging and may, therefore, theoretically be targeted without administration of intravenous contrast. Some lesions are most conspicuous in the latter contrast-enhanced phase, requiring multiple imaging cycles prior to targeting.

The equipment for the intervention requested should be prepared before a patient enters the MR imaging suite so that the procedure team can focus on patient positioning and comfort and lesion identification during image acquisition, thus enhancing intraprocedural efficiency. In cases in which multiple lesions are targeted, discussion among the procedure team members should cover not only the approach to the lesion but also the sequence of lesions to be localized.

The optimal approach to central lesions may be difficult to estimate in some cases because the breast can be distorted due to compression during the MR imaging–guided breast biopsy. The configuration of the coil and patient body habitus also influence the biopsy approach. Using grids on both sides of the breast permits access from either the medial or lateral aspect of the breast, thus ensuring the shortest or safest approach for biopsy.

Patient Preparation and Risks

The radiologist should meet with the patient to discuss the reason for the requested intervention, the events that occur during the procedure, and the composition of the procedure team. Addressing patients concerns prior to the procedure ensures greater intraprocedural compliance. The radiologist should emphasize that the patient should remain still during the procedure to avoid lengthening the procedure time and compromising targeting accuracy. The discussion should include the possibility of nonvisualization of the lesion, in which case the procedure is not feasible. The follow-up strategy in the event of nonvisualization of the lesion should also be discussed to encourage adherence with this strategy should it be needed.

The morbidity and complication rates from MR imaging–guided breast interventions are low.[19] The risks include infection, pain, bleeding, and injury to adjacent structures, which depend on lesion location and should be discussed in detail on a case-by-case basis to address the specific structures at risk.

The patient's medical records may be reviewed or a focused medical history may be performed to determine whether the patient has an increased risk of bleeding (bleeding diathesis, medications, and herbal supplements). A wide variety of herbal supplements act as coagulation inhibitors and/or potentiate the effect of antithrombotic and antiplatelet therapies.[20] Discontinuation of herbal supplements that increase the risk of bleeding is advised. For patients on anticoagulation therapies, the risk of bleeding must be weighed against the risk of thromboembolic events, such as stroke or coronary events, should anticoagulation be discontinued. Patients at high risk or intermediate risk of thromboembolic events may be referred for bridge therapy with short-acting injectable blood thinners under the supervision of the patient's treating physician. Proceeding with the intervention may be considered in patients at high risk or intermediate risk of thromboembolic events unable to undergo bridge therapy because the incidence of significant hematomas is low.[21–23]

STEPS COMMON TO ALL MR IMAGING–GUIDED BREAST INTERVENTIONS
Positioning

Optimal patient positioning requires consideration of patient size and breast size in relationship to an imaging unit's bore cavity size and coil type. Improper patient positioning results not only in breast tissue overcompression and interference with contrast enhancement but also inhomogeneous fat suppression and artifact, hindering breast cancer detection and evaluation.[24] Improper positioning may also cause pain and discomfort for a patient, resulting in patient motion artifact and inability for the patient to cooperate fully during the examination. Positioning may be challenging in patients with breathing difficulties and those with claustrophobia who may require medication to tolerate the imaging process.

Proper positioning of the breast in the coil is achieved when the breast tissue is free-hanging without skin folds or protruding abdominal tissue bulges and with nipples pointing straight without deviation.[24] To achieve this, it is critical to check arm positioning and visually check breast position from all openings of the coil, with a final check of the triplane localizer images.[24]

Targeting

After triplane localizer images, sagittal, dynamic fat-saturated T1 sequences are performed before and after administration of a gadolinium-based contrast agent. The precontrast sequence can be used to ensure the quality of fat saturation and inclusion of the area of the targeted lesion, the grid (which is a plastic panel with uniformly spaced square openings that allow access to the breast), and fiducial marker (**Figs. 1**, **2A** and **2B**).

Once the targeted lesion is identified in the appropriate MR imaging sequence, lesion coordinates are calculated. The targeted lesion may be annotated on the MR imaging console, and the annotation may be propagated to the image containing the grid and fiducial marker, allowing the radiologist to determine the optimal position of the needle guide and optimal needle entry site within the needle guide (**Fig. 2B**). Lesion depth can be estimated by counting the number of images from the skin surface where the grid is visualized to the targeted lesion and multiplying that number by the slice thickness. Alternatively, a post-contrast axial, fat-saturated T1 sequence may be performed to measure lesion depth from the overlying skin (**Fig. 2C**).

Lesion coordinates may also be determined with the use of commercially available software. The software determines the depth of the targeted lesion, the square in which the needle guide is placed within the grid, and the needle entry site within the needle guide (**Fig. 3**).

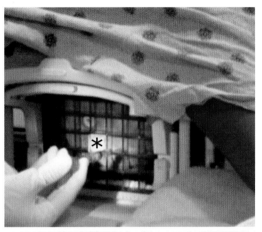

Fig. 1. Patient positioned prone for MR imaging–guided breast biopsy undergoing administration of local anesthetic. The breast is under compression by a plastic grid, which has a fiducial marker (*asterisk*) positioned away from the targeted lesion.

Lesion accessibility is determined after the lesion coordinates have been obtained. Proximity of the device (biopsy needle and clip needle or localization needle) to skin, nipple, pectoralis muscle, or breast implant may result in inadvertent injury.

Intervention

Prior to the requested intervention, the skin within the grid square chosen as the needle entry site is cleaned and anesthetized. Antisepsis is achieved with alcohol plus iodine-iodophors or chlorhexidine gluconate.[25] Local anesthesia is commonly achieved with lidocaine or bupivacaine, an amide-class anesthetic. Allergic reactions to lidocaine are rare and often related to the preservative (methylparaben) in local anesthetics. Use of a preservative-free preparation or use of an ester, like procaine or chloroprocaine, may be alternatives for patients with prior allergic reaction to lidocaine. Addition of epinephrine (1:100,000 or 1:200,000 dilution) not only aids in hemostasis but also increases the duration of anesthesia.[26] The pain associated with the administration of local anesthetics may be ameliorated by slow injection and buffering with sodium bicarbonate (8.4%). Buffering also increases dispersion of the local anesthetic through the soft tissues and hastens the onset of anesthesia.[27]

Postintervention Care

Once the intervention is finished, the breast is slowly released from the intervention coil. After a

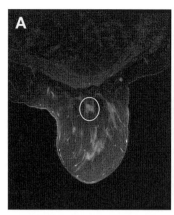
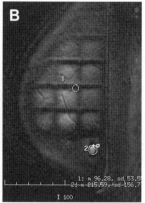
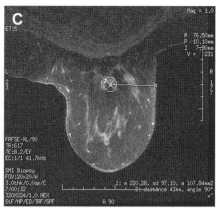

Fig. 2. Manual targeting for MR imaging–guided breast biopsy in a 52-year-old woman with a suspicious lesion detected during screening breast MR imaging. (A) Axial fat-suppressed T1-weighted postcontrast MR image demonstrates an irregular mass at the 12 o'clock position (circle). (B) Sagittal fat-suppressed T1-weighted postcontrast MR image demonstrates the grid as crossing black lines delineating squares where the needle guide may be positioned. The targeted lesion depicted as a circle (1) propagated to the image illustrating the grid. The fiducial marker (2) is a T1 hyperintense round structure placed away from the lesion (1). (C) Axial fat-suppressed T1-weighted postcontrast MR image with the lesion of interest (circle) allows precise measurement of the depth of the target (1). Fiducial marker (2) not visible in this superior image.

biopsy, hemostasis is achieved by manual pressure. The skin is then covered with sterile strips in preparation for postprocedure mammography. A compression bandage may be applied to minimize postprocedure hematomas after biopsy or clip placement.

MR IMAGING–GUIDED BIOPSY

The challenges with MR imaging–guided biopsy include lesion accessibility, decreasing lesion conspicuity over time, and confirmation of sampling adequacy.[9] For MR imaging–guided biopsy, various biopsy kits are available. The kits rely on the use of coaxial technique and contain some components that are for use only outside the magnet bore and others that are safe within the magnet bore (Fig. 4A). The nonferrous stylet is used outside the bore of the magnet to guide the introducer sheath into proper position. Numbers on the introducer sheath indicate the depth to which it may be introduced. The plastic

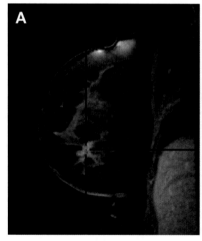
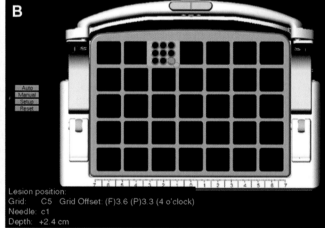

Lesion position:
Grid: C5   Grid Offset: (F)3.6 (P)3.3 (4 o'clock)
Needle: c1
Depth: +2.4 cm

Fig. 3. Computer-aided targeting in a 63-year-old woman with right breast cancer presenting with an irregular mass during staging breast MR imaging. (A) Sagittal fat-suppressed T1-weighted postcontrast MR image demonstrates an irregular mass in the right breast identified in the computer-aided detection (CAD) system (crosshairs). (B) The CAD system provides a graphic depicting the optimal entry point for the biopsy needle. Because the targeted lesion resides beneath a grid junction (open circle), the CAD system highlights an alternate entry point (colored circle). The lesion depth is calculated by the CAD system.

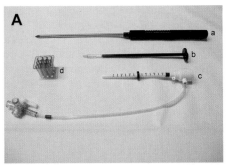
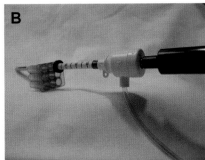
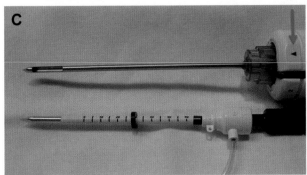
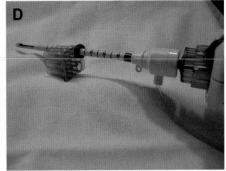

Fig. 4. MR imaging–guided breast biopsy kit components. (*A*). The kit includes (a) cutting introducer stylet, (b) plastic obturator, (c) plastic introducer sheath with numbers indicating insertion depth and a mobile stop (*black ring*), and (d) needle guide. (*B*) The needle guide may be placed prior to or in conjunction with the stylet-introducer sheath system. (*C*) Needle aperture location corresponds to a blue triangular marking on the biopsy device (*arrow*). (*D*) Biopsy needle within the introducer sheath, depicting the needle aperture in relationship to the needle guide.

obturator is placed in the introducer sheath, and the tip of the obturator is advanced to the expected location of sampling. The needle guide provides support and aids in alignment of the introducer sheath, obturator, and biopsy needle while also allowing for precision in the selection of the needle entry site.

Place the Biopsy Device

After the administration of local anesthetics, a dermatotomy (skin nick) may be made at the preference of the operator to accommodate the stylet and introducer sheath. The needle guide may be placed prior to or in conjunction with the stylet–introducer sheath system (**Fig. 4**B). The system may be advanced using a twisting or rotating motion to avoid puckering and displacement of the breast. Once the predetermined depth has been reached, the stylet is exchanged for the plastic obturator. Postcontrast MR images are then performed to confirm the appropriateness of obturator placement and delineate any corrective actions that may be needed. If further advancement is required, the plastic obturator is exchanged for the stylet, and the stylet–introducer sheath system is advanced as necessary. The stylet is exchanged for the plastic obturator when adequate placement as confirmed

with imaging is desired. Once the targeted lesion has been reached, the plastic obturator is exchanged for the biopsy device (**Fig. 4**C, D).

Sampling

Adequacy of sampling is of great importance in MR imaging–guided breast biopsies. Sampling technique depends on the relationship of the biopsy device to the target and adjacent sensitive structures like skin and pectoralis muscle. Vacuum-assisted needles allow for tissue to be pulled into the probe and also allow for real-time directional sampling.[28] Although the usual number of samples is 12 (typically 1 sample per o'clock position), additional samples may be obtained if targeting is offset.[19]

Directional sampling may be needed if the grid obscures the optimal entry site, thereby causing the needle entry to be offset to the underlying target. Directional sampling requires understanding the relationship between the needle aperture, as indicated on the biopsy device by a distinct marking, and the lesion (see **Fig. 4**C). The vacuum-assisted needle may also contain additional clock face annotations to further guide sampling. As the relationship of the clock positions to patient anatomy varies according to the breast and the approach used, familiarity with the marking that indicates the needle aperture is imperative.

Confirm the Adequacy of Sampling

Once sampling is complete, the biopsy cavity may be subjected to lavage and aspiration to minimize hematoma formation. The biopsy device is then exchanged for the obturator, and postbiopsy MR images are obtained to determine sampling adequacy. If no or little residual enhancement corresponding to the targeted lesion is identified, a marker clip may be placed via the introducer sheath to facilitate identification of the lesion if surgical resection is later deemed necessary. If the target seems unchanged, repeat sampling should be performed, followed by additional postbiopsy imaging. A rapidly developing hematoma may preclude further sampling and should prompt placement of a marker clip and management of the hematoma. Whether MR imaging is necessary after marker clip placement is controversial. The goal of such imaging is to demonstrate marker clip deployment. Postbiopsy changes may impede identification of the marker clip, however, because the signal void corresponding to the marker clip may resemble air, which is often introduced during biopsy.[9,19]

Two-view mammography, often consisting of craniocaudal and 90° views, is performed to confirm marker clip deployment. The location of the marker clip on the postbiopsy mammogram is compared with the expected location of the target based on prebiopsy MR imaging. Possible marker clip displacement is reported, and the biopsy cavity, if present as an air-filled space, is annotated on the mammogram (Fig. 5). If the marker clip does not deploy, the patient may be brought to the ultrasound suite, where the biopsy cavity may be targeted for ultrasound-guided marker clip placement (see Fig. 5).

Approach to Difficult Lesions

Several factors influence the complexity of MR imaging–guided breast biopsy, including the target location, the presence of breast implants, and the number of targets to be sampled.

Markedly posterior lesions may be difficult to access. Imaging once the patient is positioned may demonstrate that such targets are in an area above the grid, necessitating a freehand approach or needle angulation (Fig. 6).

If the lesion to be biopsied is in a breast with an implant, the implant must be displaced to minimize the risk of implant rupture and ensure the adequacy of sampling (Fig. 7).

When simultaneous biopsy of multiple targets has been requested, the biopsy supplies and equipment should be set up in advance. The vacuum-assisted devices should be available to be opened and quickly set up once the targets are visualized. It is possible that the patient may need to return for an additional day of biopsy if the number of targets to be biopsied necessitates a volume of local anesthesia that exceeds the maximum recommended dose of anesthetic used.

MR IMAGING–GUIDED CLIP PLACEMENT

MR imaging–compatible clips may be placed in conjunction with an MR imaging–guided biopsy or without a preceding biopsy. In cancer patients for whom breast-conserving surgery may be an option, MR imaging–guided clip placement of a broad area of known disease or adjacent satellites prior to neoadjuvant therapy facilitates preoperative localization at the time of surgery.

Once the target has been identified and its depth has been calculated, the clip needle may be advanced. Care must be taken to advance the needle to the proper depth because clip needles do not have distance annotations or a depth stop. Imaging with the clip needle in place is not feasible; therefore, verification of proper depth is not possible prior to clip deployment. A sterile ruler may be used to measure the proper depth on the needle. If a needle guide is used, the depth of the needle guide must be accounted for by addition of an extra 2 cm. On the postprocedure images, the signal void corresponding to the clip is used to confirm adequate clip deployment (Fig. 8). Postprocedure mammography is performed, and the location of the marker clip on the mammogram is compared with the expected location of the target based on preprocedure MR imaging.

MR IMAGING–GUIDED NEEDLE LOCALIZATION

MR imaging–guided needle localization is performed when MR imaging–guided biopsy is not feasible and surgical biopsy is needed. Once the target has been identified and its depth has been calculated, an MR imaging–compatible 20-gauge hook needle is advanced to the appropriate depth. As in the case of MR imaging–guided clip placement, if a needle guide is used, the depth of the needle guide must be accounted for by addition of an extra 2 cm. Postprocedure mammography is performed, and the location of the localization

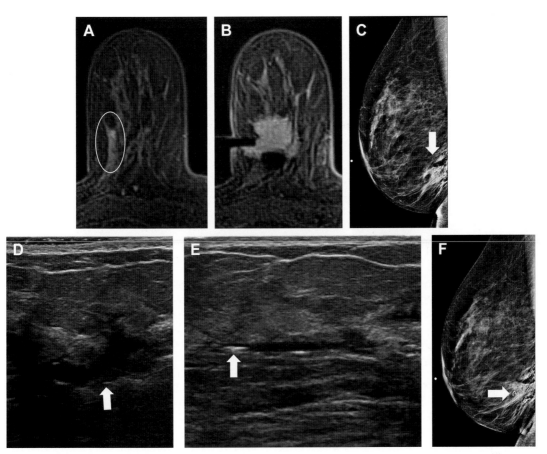

Fig. 5. Ultrasound-guided marker clip placement following MR imaging–guided biopsy in a 72-year-old woman with ILC of the left breast and unsuccessful MR imaging–guided clip placement. (*A*) Axial fat-suppressed T1-weighted postcontrast MR image demonstrates suspicious nonmass enhancement in the right breast (*oval*). (*B*) Axial fat-suppressed T1-weighted postcontrast MR image demonstrates a postbiopsy hematoma and air within the biopsy site but no clear indication of presence of marker clip. (*C*) Postprocedure mammogram demonstrates an air-filled biopsy cavity without an associated marker clip (*arrow*). (*D*) Longitudinal ultrasound image of the right breast demonstrates a hypoechoic area corresponding to the biopsy cavity (*arrow*). (*E*) Longitudinal ultrasound image of the right breast after ultrasound-guided clip deployment demonstrates a hyperechoic clip within the biopsy cavity (*arrow*). (*F*) Post–clip placement mammogram confirms deployment of the marker clip (*arrow*) within the biopsy cavity from the MR imaging–guided biopsy done the same day. Biopsy and final surgical histopathology confirmed ILC.

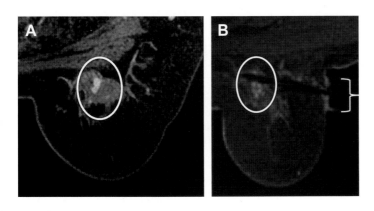

Fig. 6. MR imaging–guided biopsy with a freehand approach in a 45-year-old woman with right nipple discharge. (*A*) Axial fat-suppressed T1-weighted postcontrast MR image demonstrates an irregular mass at 12 o'clock position (*circle*). (*B*) Appearance of the targeted lesion (*circle*) may be altered at the time of biopsy. Lesion access was optimized by angulation of the needle toward the chest wall with the needle guide in place (*bracket*). Histopathology result confirmed ADH and possible DCIS.

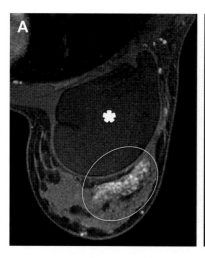

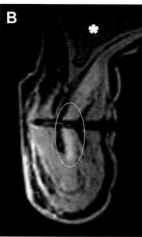

Fig. 7. MR imaging–guided biopsy with displacement of a breast implant in a 42-year-old woman with a BRCA2 mutation. (*A*) Axial fat-suppressed T1-weighted postcontrast MR image demonstrates suspicious nonmass enhancement (*circle*), anterior to implant (*asterisk*). (*B*) Axial fat-suppressed T1-weighted postcontrast MR image with implant displacement (*asterisk*) to allow biopsy access to the lesion. Implant displacement results in alteration of the appearance of the targeted lesion (*circle*). Histopathology result confirmed atypical lobular hyperplasia.

wire on the mammogram is compared with the expected location of the target based on preprocedure MR imaging (**Fig. 9**).

IMAGING-PATHOLOGY CORRELATION AFTER MR IMAGING–GUIDED BIOPSY

Because successful retrieval of the targeted lesion cannot be confirmed by visual inspection of biopsy specimens or specimen radiography, pathology review is essential. The pathology results should be in agreement with the probability of malignancy according to the BI-RADS assessment category assigned to the targeted lesion and account for the imaging findings. When the targeted lesion is a mass, the histopathology result should account for a mass-forming lesion (eg, invasive carcinoma, papilloma, fibroadenoma, lymph node, fat necrosis, or pseudoangiomatous stromal hyperplasia).[8] When the targeted lesion is nonmass enhancement, the expected histopathology results would include ductal carcinoma in situ (DCIS), invasive lobular carcinoma (ILC), periductal mastitis, fibrocystic changes, and stromal fibrosis.[7,8,11] The published rates of imaging-pathology concordance for MR imaging–guided breast biopsy range from 96% to 100%.[1–4,6,14,15]

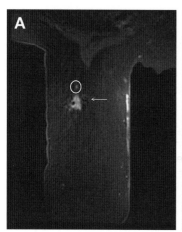

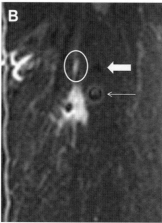

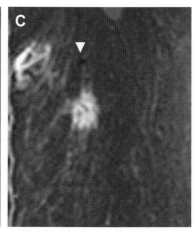

Fig. 8. MR imaging–guided marker clip placement in a 45-year-old woman with left breast cancer undergoing neoadjuvant therapy prior to breast-conserving surgery. (*A*) Axial fat-suppressed T1-weighted postcontrast MR image demonstrates an oval mass with irregular margins (*circled*) located posterior to known malignancy, consistent with satellite disease. The clip placed under ultrasound guidance (*arrow*) is located anterior and medial to the satellite lesion. MR imaging–guided clip placement was requested to delineate the extent of disease for preoperative localization and optimize breast-conserving surgery. (*B*) MR imaging–guided clip placement of posterior satellite (*circle*) (first attempt) with medial migration of the clip placed under MR imaging guidance (*thick arrow*). Note also the clip initially placed under ultrasound guidance (*thin arrow*). (*C*) Additional (second attempt) MR imaging–guided clip placement demonstrates a clip (*arrowhead*) appropriately located at the site of the targeted satellite lesion.

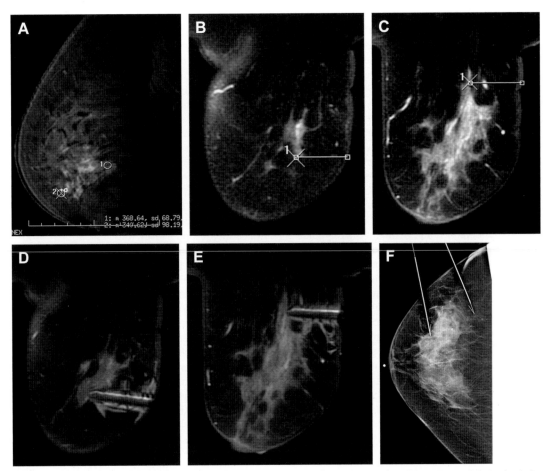

Fig. 9. MR imaging–guided needle localization of a large area of nonmass enhancement. (*A*) Sagittal fat-suppressed T1-weighted postcontrast MR image of the breast demonstrates large area of nonmass enhancement corresponding to biopsy-proved ADH. Surgical excision with MR imaging–guided 2-needle bracket localization (1, 2) was planned for additional tissue sampling. (*B*) Axial fat-suppressed T1-weighted postcontrast MR image used to measure the depth (1) of the anteroinferior extent of the nonmass enhancement. (*C*) Axial fat-suppressed T1-weighted postcontrast MR image used to measure the depth (1) of the posterosuperior extent of the nonmass enhancement. (*D*) Axial fat-suppressed T1-weighted postcontrast MR image demonstrates the needle tip at the anteroinferior extent of the nonmass enhancement. (*E*) Axial fat-suppressed T1-weighted postcontrast MR image demonstrates the needle tip at the posterosuperior extent of the nonmass enhancement. (*F*) Full-field digital mammography craniocaudal view with the 2 bracket localization needles deployed under MR imaging guidance. Final histopathology result confirmed a 6-cm area of DCIS.

After pathology review, an addendum to the biopsy report should be issued noting imaging-pathology concordance or discordance. This addendum should include final follow-up management recommendations for the referring physician and patient. When there is imaging-pathology discordance, surgical excision or repeat biopsy should be performed for definitive diagnosis. If histopathology results are malignant, recommendation for surgical management should be expeditiously communicated to the referring physician. Consultation with the pathologist is essential in discordant cases and in cases in which the pathology result indicates the presence of a high-risk lesion, which may require surgical excision.

Management of Lesions with Imaging-Concordant Benign Pathology Results

Management of MR imaging–detected breast lesions with imaging-concordant benign findings on histopathology review after MR imaging–guided biopsy is not standardized.[29,30]

Variable imaging follow-up recommendations for lesions with imaging-concordant benign histopathology results have been published including 6-month to 12-month follow-up MR imaging.[8–10,16] In 2009, Li and colleagues[31] reported a 2.3% (4/177) rate of upgrade to carcinoma in their group of suspicious MR imaging–detected breast lesions that had imaging-concordant benign results on

MR imaging–guided biopsy. These MR imaging–guided biopsy lesions were subjected to repeat biopsy or surgery because of change in size or morphology on short-term follow-up MR imaging or because of ineffective targeting at the time of MR imaging–guided biopsy.[31] This study suggested that management recommendations of lesions with imaging-concordant benign pathology may be best issued when follow-up MR imaging is performed 6 months or more after the biopsy procedure.[31] In 2017, however, Huang and colleagues[32] reported a rate of upgrade to invasive carcinoma of only 0.6% (1/169) after surgical or imaging follow-up of lesions with imaging-concordant benign result at MR imaging–guided biopsy. No biopsy targeting issues were reported in their study. These investigators concluded that with meticulous and standardized biopsy technique, MR imaging follow-up may not be needed in this group of patients. They suggested that routine annual mammographic follow-up may be sufficient for patients with imaging-concordant benign findings on MR imaging–guided biopsy.[32] Even though more studies are needed to define the standard of care for this patient population, the reported rate of missed cancers at 6 months is less than 1% across published series.[8–10,16]

Management of Lesions with Imaging-Concordant High-Risk Pathology Results

High-risk breast lesions include flat epithelial atypia (FEA), atypical ductal hyperplasia (ADH), lobular neoplasia (LN) (atypical LN and lobular carcinoma in situ), radial scar (radial sclerosing lesion, scleroelastotic lesion, sclerosing papillary lesion, and complex sclerosing lesion), papillary lesion (benign or atypical), and mucocele-like lesions. Management of imaging-concordant high-risk findings on histopathology review after MR imaging–guided biopsy is not standardized. Surgical excision of these lesions is often recommended because of the possibility for upgrade to malignancy at surgery and the significant subjectivity in the pathologic interpretation of such lesions.[33]

Studies to date on rates of upgrade to malignancy (invasive carcinoma or DCIS) for MR imaging–guided biopsy lesions with high-risk histopathology are limited by their retrospective design and small sample size.[34–39] There is also lack of uniformity among studies regarding the definition of a high-risk lesion, and many studies do not report on papillomas, FEA, and mucocele-like lesions. For LN, many studies make no distinction between atypical lobular hyperplasia and lobular carcinoma in situ.

Upgrade rates to malignancy are 31% to 50% for ADH and 5.6% to 50% for LN when diagnosed by MR imaging–guided biopsy.[34–38] In these studies, ADH cases were upgraded to DCIS, invasive ductal carcinoma (IDC), and invasive mixed ductal-lobular carcinoma. Similarly, the LN cases were upgraded to DCIS, invasive carcinoma not otherwise specified, IDC, and ILC.[34,35,37,38]

Upgrade rates to malignancy are 0% to 24% for radial scars and 0% to 40% for FEA.[34,35,37–39] When upgrade to malignancy occurred in the cases of radial scar, final diagnoses were DCIS, invasive tubular carcinoma, and IDC.[35,37] Tozaki and colleagues[39] found that 5 of 102 lesions studied (5%) were FEA, and 2 of these (40%) were upgraded to malignancy. In contrast, Crystal and colleagues[34] and Heller and colleagues[35] found that only 2 of 161 lesions studied (1.0%) and 16 of 1145 lesions (1.4%), were FEA, and none was upgraded to malignancy.

In the 2 studies that classified papillary lesions as high-risk rather than benign lesions, malignancy upgrade rates were reported to be 5.9% and 6.7%. The lesions were upgraded to DCIS and IDC on surgical excision.[35,37] No study has reported the frequency and malignancy upgrade rates for mucocele-like lesions at MR imaging–guided biopsy.

For patients with high-risk histopathology at MR imaging–guided biopsy, an individualized management plan, tailored to the patient and the specific lesion type, may be arrived at by a multidisciplinary team approach. The team, which includes primary care, radiology, pathology, and surgery, should rigorously review the diagnostic imaging studies, the biopsy images, and the extent of the lesion on pathology so that a group consensus can be reached on an appropriate plan of care for the patient.[17] Because there are currently few published reports on the outcome of high-risk breast lesions detected on MR imaging–guided biopsy, more studies are needed to determine the optimal management for these high-risk lesions.

SUMMARY

MR imaging–guided interventions, including percutaneous biopsy, clip placement, and preoperative needle localization, are safe, accurate, and effective. These have become integral to breast imaging practices due to greater utilization of breast MR imaging. The various interventions discussed in this article allow for percutaneous diagnosis of breast lesions and aid surgical approach when excision is needed. As with breast biopsies performed under other guidance modalities, imaging-pathology correlation after MR imaging–guided biopsy is essential to confirm accuracy of sampling and guide creation of a multidisciplinary management plan.

REFERENCES

1. Han BK, Schnall MD, Orel SG, et al. Outcome of MRI-guided breast biopsy. AJR Am J Roentgenol 2008;191(6):1798–804.

2. Mahoney MC. Initial clinical experience with a new MRI vacuum-assisted breast biopsy device. J Magn Reson Imaging 2008;28(4):900–5.

3. Abe H, Schmidt RA, Shah RN, et al. MR-directed ("Second-Look") ultrasound examination for breast lesions detected initially on MRI: MR and sonographic findings. AJR Am J Roentgenol 2010; 194(2):370–7.

4. Spick C, Baltzer PA. Diagnostic utility of second-look US for breast lesions identified at MR imaging: systematic review and meta-analysis. Radiology 2014; 273(2):401–9.

5. Kuhl CK, Strobel K, Bieling H, et al. Impact of preoperative breast MR imaging and MR-guided surgery on diagnosis and surgical outcome of women with invasive breast cancer with and without DCIS component. Radiology 2017;284(3):645–55.

6. Orel SG, Rosen M, Mies C, et al. MR imaging-guided 9-gauge vacuum-assisted core-needle breast biopsy: initial experience. Radiology 2006; 238(1):54–61.

7. Dogan BE, Le-Petross CH, Stafford JR, et al. MRI-guided vacuum-assisted breast biopsy performed at 3 T with a 9-gauge needle: preliminary experience. AJR Am J Roentgenol 2012;199(5):W651–3.

8. Gao Y, Bagadiya NR, Jardon ML, et al. Outcomes of preoperative MRI-guided needle localization of non-palpable mammographically occult breast lesions. AJR Am J Roentgenol 2016;207(3):676–84.

9. Liberman L, Bracero N, Morris E, et al. MRI-guided 9-gauge vacuum-assisted breast biopsy: initial clinical experience. AJR Am J Roentgenol 2005;185(1): 183–93.

10. Liberman L, Morris EA, Dershaw DD, et al. Fast MRI-guided vacuum-assisted breast biopsy: initial experience. AJR Am J Roentgenol 2003;181(5):1283–93.

11. Perlet C, Heinig A, Prat X, et al. Multicenter study for the evaluation of a dedicated biopsy device for MR-guided vacuum biopsy of the breast. Eur Radiol 2002;12(6):1463–70.

12. Fischer U, Vosshenrich R, Döler W, et al. MR imaging-guided breast intervention: experience with two systems. Radiology 1995;195(2):533–8.

13. Heywang-Köbrunner SH, Heinig A, Pickuth D, et al. Interventional MRI of the breast: lesion localisation and biopsy. Eur Radiol 2000;10(1):36–45.

14. Patriciu A, Chen M, Iranpanah B, et al. A tissue stabilization device for MRI-guided breast biopsy. Med Eng Phys 2014;36(9):1197–204.

15. DeMartini WB, Rahbar H. Breast magnetic resonance imaging technique at 1.5 T and 3 T: requirements for quality imaging and American College of Radiology accreditation. Magn Reson Imaging Clin N Am 2013;21(3):475–82.

16. D'Orsi CJ, Sickles EA, Mendelson EB, et al. ACR BI-RADS® atlas, breast imaging reporting and data system. Reston (VA): American College of Radiology; 2013.

17. Park VY, Kim MJ, Kim EK, et al. Second-look US: how to find breast lesions with a suspicious MR imaging appearance. Radiographics 2013;33(5): 1361–75.

18. Telegrafo M, Rella L, Stabile Ianora AA, et al. Supine breast US: how to correlate breast lesions from prone MRI. Br J Radiol 2016;89(1059):20150497.

19. Plantade R, Thomassin-Naggara I. MRI vacuum-assisted breast biopsies. Diagn Interv Imaging 2014;95(9):779–801.

20. Wong WW, Gabriel A, Maxwell GP, et al. Bleeding risks of herbal, homeopathic, and dietary supplements: a hidden nightmare for plastic surgeons? Aesthet Surg J 2012;32(3):332–46.

21. Chetlen AL, Kasales C, Mack J, et al. Hematoma formation during breast core needle biopsy in women taking antithrombotic therapy. AJR Am J Roentgenol 2013;201(1):215–22.

22. du Breuil AL, Umland EM. Outpatient management of anticoagulation therapy. Am Fam Physician 2007;75(7):1031–42.

23. Manchikanti L, Falco FJ, Benyamin RM, et al. Assessment of bleeding risk of interventional techniques: a best evidence synthesis of practice patterns and perioperative management of anticoagulant and antithrombotic therapy. Pain Physician 2013;16(2 Suppl):SE261–318.

24. Yeh ED, Georgian-Smith D, Raza S, et al. Positioning in breast MR imaging to optimize image quality. Radiographics 2014;34(1):E1–17.

25. Darouiche RO, Wall MJ Jr, Itani KM, et al. Chlorhexidine-Alcohol versus povidone-iodine for surgical-site antisepsis. N Engl J Med 2010;362(1):18–26.

26. Achar S, Kundu S. Principles of office anesthesia: part I. Infiltrative anesthesia. Am Fam Physician 2002;66(1):91–4.

27. Scarfone RJ, Jasani M, Gracely EJ. Pain of local anesthetics: rate of administration and buffering. Ann Emerg Med 1998;31(1):36–40.

28. Parker SH, Klaus AJ. Performing a breast biopsy with a directional, vacuum-assisted biopsy instrument. Radiographics 1997;17(5):1233–52.

29. Huang ML, Adrada BE, Candelaria R, et al. Stereotactic breast biopsy: pitfalls and pearls. Tech Vasc Interv Radiol 2014;17(1):32–9.

30. Huang ML, Hess K, Candelaria RP, et al. Comparison of the accuracy of US-guided biopsy of breast masses performed with 14-gauge, 16-gauge and 18-gauge automated cutting needle biopsy devices, and review of the literature. Eur Radiol 2017;27(7): 2928–33.

31. Li J, Dershaw DD, Lee CH, et al. MRI follow-up after concordant, histologically benign diagnosis of breast lesions sampled by MRI-guided biopsy. AJR Am J Roentgenol 2009;193(3):850–5.

32. Huang ML, Speer M, Dogan BE, et al. Imaging-concordant benign MRI-guided vacuum-assisted breast biopsy may not warrant MRI follow-up. AJR Am J Roentgenol 2017;208(4):916–22.

33. Krishnamurthy S, Bevers T, Kuerer H, et al. Multidisciplinary considerations in the management of high-risk breast lesions. AJR Am J Roentgenol 2012; 198(2):W132–40.

34. Crystal P, Sadaf A, Bukhanov K, et al. High-risk lesions diagnosed at MRI-guided vacuum-assisted breast biopsy: can underestimation be predicted? Eur Radiol 2011;21(3):582–9.

35. Heller SL, Elias K, Gupta A, et al. Outcome of high-risk lesions at MRI-guided 9-gauge vacuum-assisted breast biopsy. AJR Am J Roentgenol 2014;202(1):237–45.

36. Liberman L, Holland AE, Marjan D, et al. Underestimation of atypical ductal hyperplasia at MRI-guided 9-gauge vacuum-assisted breast biopsy. AJR Am J Roentgenol 2007;188(3):684–90.

37. Lourenco AP, Khalil H, Sanford M, et al. High-risk lesions at MRI-guided breast biopsy: frequency and rate of underestimation. AJR Am J Roentgenol 2014;203(3):682–6.

38. Rauch GM, Dogan BE, Smith TB, et al. Outcome analysis of 9-gauge MRI-guided vacuum-assisted core needle breast biopsies. AJR Am J Roentgenol 2012;198(2):292–9.

39. Tozaki M, Yamashiro N, Sakamoto M, et al. Magnetic resonance-guided vacuum-assisted breast biopsy: results in 100 Japanese women. Jpn J Radiol 2010;28(7):527–33.

Developments in Breast Imaging
Update on New and Evolving MR Imaging and Molecular Imaging Techniques

Samantha Lynn Heller, MD, PhD, Laura Heacock, MD,
Linda Moy, MD*

KEYWORDS

- MR imaging • 3-T • Diffusion-weighted imaging • Abbreviated MR imaging
- Molecular breast imaging • Breast-specific γ-imaging • Positron emission mammography
- 18F-FDG PET

KEY POINTS

- The 3-T field strength MR imaging offers an increase in both temporal and spatial resolution over lower magnet strengths.
- Diffusion-weighted imaging is a short sequence that does not require contrast; it increases breast specificity and improves characterization of breast lesions as benign or malignant.
- Growing evidence shows that a shortened MR imaging examination could offer a high sensitivity for cancer detection with broader applicability than current MR imaging screening protocols.
- Molecular imaging techniques offer high sensitivity for cancer detection across breast densities, although relatively high radiation doses with these technologies must be taken into account.
- PET/MR imaging offers the potential of combining functional and anatomic imaging, directed to the breast and the rest of the body in the context of breast cancer staging.

INTRODUCTION

There have been exciting and varied developments in the field of breast imaging in recent years, developments encompassing multiple modalities with the promise of improving cancer detection. In addition to improved technological capabilities (such as higher magnetic field strengths), there has been growing interest in broader applicability for the breast MR imaging screening examination. In addition, there has been focus on and consideration for the additive impact that functional—in addition to anatomic—analysis of breast pathology have on better identifying and characterizing breast lesions; these developments apply both to the field of MR imaging (multiparametric approaches, including diffusion-weighted imaging [DWI]) and to the field

of nuclear medicine (breast-specific γ-imaging [BSGI], positron emission mammography [PEM], and PET with fludeoxyglucose F 18/MR imaging [PET/MR imaging]), all of which are reviewed in this article. This article reviews these evolving breast imaging techniques with attention to the strengths, weaknesses, and applications of these varied approaches to breast imaging. In doing so, we hope to give the reader familiarity with the state of current developments in the field and to increase awareness of what to expect in future years in the field of breast imaging.

MR IMAGING

MR imaging of the breast has become a mainstay of breast imaging, both in the diagnostic realm

Disclosure Statement: The authors have no disclosures.
NYU School of Medicine, NYU Laura and Isaac Perlmutter Cancer Center, 3rd Floor, New York, NY 10016, USA
* Corresponding author.
E-mail address: Linda.Moy@nyumc.org

Magn Reson Imaging Clin N Am 26 (2018) 247–258
https://doi.org/10.1016/j.mric.2017.12.003

(extent of disease, implant evaluation, workup of unknown primary in the context of axillary lymphadenopathy) and in the screening realm (high-risk women and, in certain cases, intermediate-risk women).[1]

Magnetic Field Strength: 3 T Versus 1.5 T

MR imaging protocol at 3 T

To allow for adequate spatial and temporal resolution, breast MR imaging should be performed at 1.0 T or greater field strength. We perform our MR imaging examinations using a 3 T magnet (TIM Trio, Siemens Medical Solutions, Erlangen, Germany) with the patient in prone positioning using a dedicated surface breast coil (Sentinelle 16 channel coil, Invivo, Gainesville, FL). Our standard imaging protocol includes a localizing sequence followed by axial T2-weighted sequence (TR/TE, 7220/84), an axial T1-weighted non–fat-suppressed 3-dimensional fast spoiled gradient-recalled echo sequence (TR/TE, 4.01/1.52; flip angle, 12°; matrix, 384 × 384; field of view, 270 mm; section thickness, 1 mm) followed by the same axial T1-weighted fat-suppressed 3-dimensional fast spoiled gradient-recalled echo sequence performed before and 3 times immediately after a rapid bolus injection of 0.1 mmol/kg of gadopentetate dimeglumine (Gadovist, Bayer Healthcare, Whippany NJ) per kilogram of body weight at an injection rate of 2.0 mL/s via an intravenous catheter followed by a saline flush. The first contrast-enhanced dynamic image corresponds with approximately 100 seconds after injection. The total duration of the dynamic study is approximately 7 minutes. After the examination, subtraction images are obtained by subtraction of the precontrast images.

Advantages of 3 T imaging

Breast imaging at 3 T allows for an increase in both temporal and spatial resolution over lower magnet strengths. Signal-to-noise ratio (SNR) improves linearly with increasing field strength. This improvement in SNR offers the potential for a faster imaging time and increased spatial resolution, although real-time factors yield an SNR that is usually 1.6 to 1.8 times the SNR at 1.5 T, rather than the theoretically expected doubled SNR.[2] The 3 T strength also offers better fat suppression (although B0 homogeneity may be more difficult at 3 T) because there is increased spectral separation of fat and water resonance at higher field strengths. The more homogenous and more effective fat suppression should translate into increased lesion conspicuity.

It is possible that 3 T is especially effective in conjunction with parallel imaging, a technique that uses decreased sampling of k space lines enabling reduced phase encoding steps by an acceleration factor R; this in turn allows for decreased acquisition times by a factor of 1.5 to 3.0,[3] with excellent spatial resolution.[4,5]

There are multiple studies demonstrating excellent lesion detection at 3 T with high sensitivity,[6,7] but it is difficult to quantify definitively the clinical value of breast MR imaging at 3 T versus 1.5 T, in particular because differences in coils and scan parameters complicate meaningful comparisons.[8] One prospective study looked at 31 women with known malignant and benign lesions who had a 1.5 T breast MR imaging scan followed by a 3 T scan 24 to 48 hours later; the authors found improved lesion conspicuity of both benign and malignant lesions at 3 T versus 1.5 T; however, this difference did not achieve significance.[9]

Disadvantages of 3 T imaging

There are potential disadvantages at higher magnetic field strengths: both chemical shift and susceptibility artifacts may be more evident at 3 T compared with 1.5 T. In addition, the energy deposited into tissue at 3 T is approximately 4 times greater at 3 T compared with 1.5 T,[2] because radiofrequency energy increases exponentially with field strength. For this reason, there is a greater risk of tissue heating and burns at higher magnetic field strengths. To maintain the specific absorption rate, the US Food and Drug Administration mandated limits (4 W/kg averaged over the body for 15 minutes),[10] protocol changes such as decreasing slices per TR, decreasing flip angle, and longer a TR may need to be used. However, such changes come at the expense of decreased SNR, tissue contrast, and breast coverage. In addition, hardware and implants that are compatible with 1.5 T systems may not be safe at 3 T. If there is any concern for patient safety in the context of a 3 T magnet, the study should be performed on a 1.5 T magnet instead. Finally, it is worth noting that although a 3 T magnet costs more than a 1.5 T magnet, billing is the same for both field strengths.

Diffusion-Weighted Imaging

DWI operates through exploiting the molecular diffusion of water through tissue. The mobility of the water molecules is altered by factors such as tissue cellularity; the degree of tissue cellularity and membrane integrity impacts water diffusion with resultant signal changes. Thus, DWI has the ability to improve breast cancer detection when the cellular structure alters owing to cancer histologic make-up. Because DWI does not require a contrast agent and is a relatively rapid sequence, often taking only 2 to 3 minutes,[11] DWI is a relatively easy addition to the standard contrast-enhanced MR imaging examination.

Technical considerations

DWI usually uses a spin echo sequence with diffusion gradient pulses and a 180° refocusing pulse. A b-value—the degree of diffusion weighting—impacts how sensitive the diffusion sequence is to water molecule mobility. The apparent diffusion coefficient (ADC) is calculated from the signal intensities at distinct b-values and can be used as a qualitative visual map and also as a quantitative means of assessing restricted diffusion. The varied range of b-values used across DWI studies has made it difficult to standardize ADC values for characterizing lesions. In our practice, we use b-values of 0 and 800. However, a metaanalysis evaluating the accuracy of DWI for breast lesion characterization based on the b-value consisting of 26 studies found that overall median ADC values were significant higher ($P<.001$) for b-values of 600 s/mm or less,[3] but that sensitivity and specificity in both groups was similar (sensitivity 91% and 89%, $P = .495$; specificity 75% and 84%, $P = .237$). Benign versus malignant characterization was best (58.4%) at a combination of b = 0 and 1000 s/mm.[3,12]

Clinical use

In conjunction with dynamic contrast-enhanced (DCE) MR imaging, DWI has been shown to increase breast specificity and to improve characterization of breast lesions as benign or malignant. A metaanalysis of 14 studies (1140 patients with 1276 breast lesions) determined that combined DWI and DCE MR imaging had better diagnostic accuracy than either DCE MR imaging or DWI alone (pooled sensitivity and specificity of 91.6% and 85.5% for combined approach vs 93.2% and 71.1% for DCE MR imaging and 86.0% and 75.6% for DWI alone). The area under the summary receiver operator characteristic curve was 0.94 for the combined protocol versus 0.85 for DCE MR imaging alone.[2] A retrospective study of 101 patients and 104 lesions found that the additional application of DWI would have avoided 29 false-positive biopsies (34.5%) by using an ADC threshold value of 1.58 × 10^{-3} mm^2/s to identify benign lesions versus malignant lesions with a lower value ADC.[13]

DWI also has shown promise for predicting biologically more significant cancers; lower ADC values have been found to correlate with indicators of aggressiveness such as Ki-67 and tumor subtype.[8,14,15]

Along similar lines, there are some recent small studies investigating the ability of DWI to differentiate between ductal carcinoma in situ (DCIS) grades and also to identify the malignant likelihood of high-risk lesions at upgrade. Using a model incorporating distinct DCE and DWI properties, Rahbar and colleagues[8] found that low-grade DCIS had lower normalized ADCs ($P = .04$) than high-grade DCIS. A recent prospective study evaluated whether ADC coefficient values could predict high-risk lesion upgrade at excision.[14] The authors identified 23 high-risk lesions, of which 6 were upgraded at surgery. These 6 high-risk lesions demonstrated significantly lower ADC than those that did not ($P = .046$). A model incorporating both lesion size and ADC provided best performance for predicting upgrade (area under the receiver operator characteristic curve of 0.89).[14] Although larger studies need to be performed, both of these studies suggest that DWI may be able to help identify those lesions that are more likely to be clinically significant.

Monitoring neoadjuvant chemotherapy

DWI has the potential to help monitor and even predict response to neoadjuvant chemotherapy in the context of treating known breast cancer. A recent retrospective study consisting of 111 patients with invasive breast cancer examined the DWI characteristics of tumors before and after treatment.[15] The mean ADC ratio (mean posttreatment ADC/mean pretreatment ADC) was significantly increased when pathologic complete response was achieved in triple-negative and HER2-positive tumors. Out of a metareview of 57 neoadjuvant treatment response studies with 5811 cases, 8 (539 cases) included DWI.[16] Although the DWI sample size was small, DWI showed high sensitivity (0.79; 0.68–0.88) for detecting pathologic complete response relative to DCE-MR imaging (0.61; 0.31–0.79).[16]

Finally, the American College of Radiology Imaging Network (ACRIN) 6698 multiinstitutional substudy of the Investigation of Serial Studies (I-SPY 2) is intended to evaluate DWI MR imaging biomarkers for assessment of breast cancer response to neoadjuvant treatment. ACRIN 6698 aims to determine if diffusion-weighted MR imaging is effective for measuring breast tumor response to neoadjuvant treatment and if response measured by DWI early in the course of taxane-based therapy is predictive of pathologic response.[17]

Evaluation of the axilla

There has been interest in determining whether DWI may help to predict metastatic lymph nodes in the context of known breast cancer; however, results are mixed to date. Kim and colleagues[18] in a retrospective study of 253 axillae found that a combination of DCE MR imaging and DWI features were helpful in predicting axillary nodal involvement with lower ADC values in malignant nodes and a high specificity (90.1%) for multiple combined features. Razek and colleagues[19] also found that combined DCE and DWI features were able to predict metastatic nodal disease in a prospective study of 34 patients with known breast cancer with statistically significant lower ADC values in involved nodes. In contrast, Rahbar and colleagues[20] found that quantitative features—including DWI parameters—of morphologically suspicious axillary lymph nodes were generally not helpful in predicting malignancy.

Abbreviated MR Imaging

As described, breast MR imaging is well-established as a tool for screening women with a known high lifetime risk of developing breast cancer. There have also been multiple investigations into whether women of intermediate lifetime risk of developing breast cancer may also benefit from MR imaging screening; several studies have suggest that women with a personal history of breast cancer or women with a history of a high-risk lesion may also benefit from annual screening.[21,22] Increasingly, the question of whether MR imaging screening should be more widely used for women of average or only slightly increased risk has become of increasing interest with evidence to suggest that MR imaging may have benefit in these women.[23] In particular, there has been increased attention to how best to image women with dense breasts (who are both at a slightly elevated lifetime risk of developing breast cancer and whose mammograms are known to be less sensitive for detection of disease); it is possible that MR imaging with its known high sensitivity for cancer detection may be an effective imaging strategy in this group. However, MR imaging is currently expensive and time consuming, with a typical examination taking 30 to 45 minutes. In the last few years, with this in mind, an increasing number of studies have been published investigating the possibility of creating a faster and less costly MR imaging breast imaging protocol that could have far broader applicability—so-called abbreviated MR imaging studies (AB-MR imaging).

Abbreviated MR Imaging protocols

A variety of abbreviated protocols have been evaluated in the literature (Table 1); protocol design operates on the principle that the increased angiogenesis and consequent rapid wash-in and wash-out of blood flow to malignant lesions will result in a rapid uptake of contrast at the first dynamic postcontrast time point. In addition, background parenchymal enhancement, which usually follows a persistent delayed kinetic pattern,[21] is least obtrusive at this same first time point. Theoretically, then, we should be able to identify cancers at the early temporal phase of the MR imaging examination without needing to incorporate the later postcontrast time points that are a part of the traditional MR imaging breast protocol (Figs. 1 and 2).

Table 1
Abbreviated imaging protocols

Study	Prospective or Retrospective	T	N	Protocol[a]	Readers (n)	Lesions
Kuhl et al,[24] 2014	P	1.5	606	Pre, post, sub, MIP	2	M, B
Mango et al,[25] 2015	R	1.5/3.0	100	Pre, post, sub, MIP	4	M
Grimm et al,[26] 2015	R	1.5/3.0	48	1. Pre, post, sub, T2 2. Pre, post, post2, sub, T2	3	M, B
Heacock et al,[27] 2016	R	3.0	107	1. Pre, post, sub 2. Pre, post, sub (priors) 3. Pre, post, sub, T2 (priors)	3	M
Harvey et al,[28] 2016	P	—	568	Pre, post, sub, MIP	—	M, B
Moschetta et al,[29] 2016	R	1.5	470	Pre, post, sub, MIP, T2, STIR	2	M, B
Bickelhaupt et al,[30] 2016	P	1.5	50	1. DWIBS, DWIBS-MIP, T2 2. Pre, post, sub, MIP, T2	2	M, B
McDonald et al,[31] 2016	R	1.5/3.0	48	Pre, DWI, ADC, T2	3	M, B
Machida et al,[32] 2017	R	3.0	88	Pre, post	2	M, B
Chen et al,[33] 2017	R	3.0	478	Sub, MIP	2	M, B
Panigrahi et al,[34] 2017	P	1.5/3.0	651	Pre, post, sub, MIP	1[a]	M, B

Abbreviations: ADC, apparent diffusion coefficient; B, benign; DWI, diffusion-weighted imaging; M, malignant; MIP, maximum intensity projection; P, prospective; post, postcontrast; pre, precontrast; R, retrospective; sub, subtraction images.
[a] Although multiple readers participated, each study was read by a single reader.

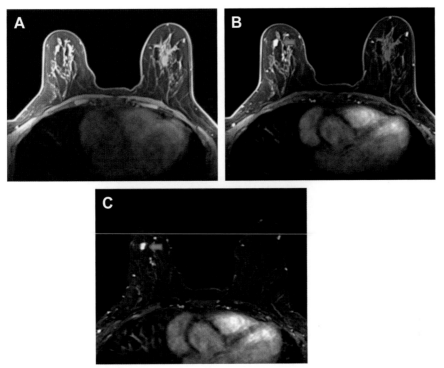

Fig. 1. A 61-year-old BRCA2-positive woman for high-risk screening using an abbreviated MR imaging protocol at 3T field strength. Mammographically and sonographically occult right breast invasive ductal carcinoma (*block arrow*) is not seen on T1-weighted precontrast images (*A*), but enhances on first T1-weighted postcontrast (*B*) and corresponding subtraction images (*C*).

To date, the studies examining abbreviated MR imaging have generally incorporated precontrast images and between 1 and 2 postcontrast images as well as accompanying subtraction images with an acquisition time of as low as 2 minutes 20 seconds.[24–27] The available work most frequently assesses an enriched cancer cohort or a high-risk screening population. Overall sensitivity and specificity of AB-MR imaging for cancer detection in this literature varies widely with a sensitivity range of 45% to 100% and specificity of 45% to 94%, suggesting the need for further studies.

There is current variability in the protocols in the literature and more work needs to be done to determine the optimal combination of sequences for cancer detection and for a screening protocol specifically. Several studies have included maximum intensity projection images[24,25,28–30] and some studies have also included T2-weighted imaging (T2-weighted images may increase reader confidence, but at the expense of additional scan time).[27,31] There has also been interest in performing high temporal resolution imaging techniques for obtaining 3-dimensional whole breast images (ultrafast MR imaging), which would allow for an abbreviated examination with kinetic analytical capability, using only a 7-second acquisition time in a recent study.[30]

There has also been increasing interest in an MR imaging abbreviated examination, which could be performed without contrast. Bickelhaupt and colleagues,[30] for example, in a prospective study of 50 patients with 24 cancers, compared an abbreviated MR imaging protocol consisting of maximum intensity projections from DWI with background suppression and also unenhanced morphologic sequences to an abbreviated contrast material-enhanced MR imaging protocol. The authors found the diffusion protocol had a sensitivity of 0.92 (95% confidence interval [CI], 0.73–0.98) and a specificity of 0.94 (95% CI, 0.77–0.99) compared with a sensitivity of 0.85 (95% CI, 0.78–0.95) and a specificity of 0.90 (95% CI, 0.72–0.97) with the contrast protocol. Another recent feasibility study evaluated full-coverage, sensitivity encoding-accelerated breast high spatial and spectral resolution MR imaging in 16 women with biopsy-proven cancer or suspicious lesions and 13 normal volunteers. The examination was 4 times faster than conventional acquisition time and offered excellent fat suppression compared with T1-weighted images, as well as higher SNR in the axilla.[10]

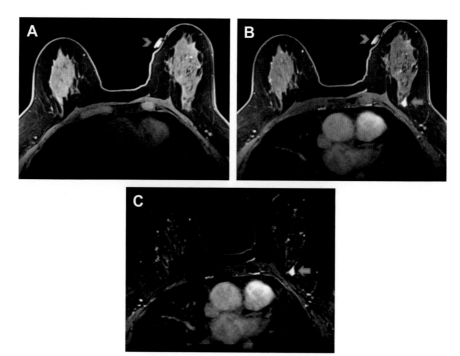

Fig. 2. A 66-year-old woman with a history of bilateral atypical lobular hyperplasia (ALH) and dense breasts imaged with abbreviated MR imaging protocol at 3T field strength. Mammographically and sonographically occult posterior left breast irregular mass (*block arrow*) is not seen on T1-weighted precontrast images (*A*), but demonstrates conspicuous enhancement on first T1 postcontrast (*B*) and subtraction images (*C*). MR imaging-guided biopsy yielded invasive lobular carcinoma. Left medial breast vitamin E marker (*chevron*) is at site of prior left breast excisional biopsy for ALH.

Because lesions that are seen on AB-MR imaging are, by definition, those with early rapid avid contrast enhancement, studies have consistently noted that lower grade invasive cancers and DCIS are less likely to be seen. In general, MR imaging has been shown to be more likely to identify invasive rather than in situ disease[35] and, for example, 60% of the lesions not seen were DCIS in a study by Mango and colleagues.[25] Early work thus raises the possibility that the cancers that are missed by AB-MR imaging may be less biologically significant cancers; however, more investigation remains to be done in this area. Lesion location also seems to have an impact on cancer detection on AB-MR imaging; for example, axillary lesions have presented challenges on several studies,[25,27] as have chest wall lesions.[26] Artifacts such as susceptibility-weighted artifacts from biopsy marker clips have also been shown to interfere with lesion conspicuity.[25,31]

Upcoming clinical trials and future directions

An Eastern Cooperative Oncology Group-American College of Radiology Imaging Network (ECOG-ACRIN) Cancer Research Group randomized phase II trial study is currently recruiting; the goal of this study is to evaluate the diagnostic accuracy of screening with abbreviated breast MR imaging compared with digital tomosynthesis mammography in detecting cancer in women with dense breasts. The findings from this trial will be particularly welcome in terms of evaluating AB-MR imaging within a screening population.[36]

Molecular Imaging Techniques

Molecular imaging of the breast offers the possibility of functional evaluation of disease states. BSGI uses technetium 99m (^{99m}Tc)-sestamibi uptake to detect increased blood flow to cancer cells. PEM is a high-resolution breast-specific gamma imaging that uses 18-fluorodeoxyglucose to evaluate molecular metabolic activity. Both technologies have higher resolution than PET/computed tomography (CT) and are, therefore, able to identify small tumors (<1 cm) that would not be visualized with PET/CT. PET/MR is another molecular imaging modality that allows the functional capabilities of nuclear medicine to be harnessed to the anatomic and multiparametric strengths of MR imaging.

Breast-specific γ-imaging

BSGI has been shown to have high sensitivity in terms of cancer detection (85.7%–96.0%) with lower specificity (60%–77%).[37,38] BSGI has also been shown to be sensitive across breast densities.[37,38] Rechtman and colleagues[38] found that BSGI was equally sensitive for breast cancer detection in nondense and dense breasts with sensitivities of 95.8% (nondense) and 95.1% (dense; $P = .459$). BSGI may be less sensitive for smaller tumors, however.[37,39] Meissnitzer and colleagues[39] found that sensitivity for lesions less than 1.0 cm decreased significantly to 60%.

BSGI also has been shown to have additive value in screening.[40] Brem and colleagues evaluated the incremental cancer detection in women at increased risk for breast cancer with negative mammograms. Of 849 patients, there were 14 BSGI-detected mammographically occult breast cancers, which is an incremental yield of 16.5 cancers per 1000 women screened. Similarly, a retrospective study of 1696 women with dense breasts and negative mammograms who underwent screening with 300 MBq (8 mCi) (99m)Tc-sestamibi[41] identified 13 mammographically occult malignancies, of which 11 were invasive with an incremental cancer detection rate of 7.7% (95% CI, 4.5%–13.1%), and a recall rate of 8.4% (95% CI, 7.2%–9.8%).

However, one of the disadvantages of gamma imaging is the increased amount of radiation exposure in comparison with mammography; this factor must be considered in any analysis of gamma imaging, in particular when considering BSGI as a breast cancer screening technique. Even though low-dose gamma imaging (7–10 mCi) has been shown to be equivalent to higher dose imaging (15–30 mCi) in terms of sensitivity and negative predictive value,[42] the overall benefit to risk ratio does not hold up favorably when compared with mammography from a radiation exposure perspective. In a study comparing benefit-to-radiation risk ratios of mammography alone, BSGI alone, and mammography plus BSGI performed annually over 10-year age intervals from ages 40 to 79 years, this unfavorable benefit to risk ration remained the case even for lower dose BSGI.[43]

Positron emission mammography
PEM uses a pair of dedicated gamma radiation detectors placed above and below the breast and mild breast compression to detect coincident gamma rays after administration of fluorine-18 fluorodeoxyglucose (18F-FDG). The breast is compressed between the detector plate and a compression paddle and mediolateral oblique and craniocaudal views are obtained as in conventional mammography. Prone PEM scanners are also available.[44]

FDG-PEM has been shown to have high diagnostic accuracy for breast cancer, including DCIS[45] with sensitivities reported at 90% to 96%

and specificities of 84% to 91%.[45–47] Like BSGI, PEM may be particularly effective in women with dense breasts. PEM has also been shown to have high sensitivity and higher specificity compared with MR imaging in assessing the extent of disease, both in the ipsilateral and the contralateral breast.[47,48]

There are limited data regarding the use of PEM in a screening context. Additionally, there are practical difficulties in using PEM as a screening modality: radiation dose, the 4- to 6-hour fast generally recommended before 18F-FDG injection to allow greater radionuclide uptake, and the need for the patient to be rested and at an optimal temperature. Nevertheless, a single-center audit of 265 women (an opportunistic screening population) reports a recall rate of 8.3% and a cancer detection rate of 2.3%.[49]

As with BSGI, consideration of using PEM must also take radiation dose into account and overcoming the higher radiation exposure of this technology compared with other breast imaging modalities remains challenging.[50] MacDonald and colleagues[50] looked at a reduced F-FDG injection activity on interpretation of PEM images and compared image interpretation between 2 postinjection imaging times (60 and 120 minutes). They evaluated 30 patients, one-half of whom underwent the standard protocol and one-half of whom received one-half of the standard activity. The authors found that reducing the image counts relative to the standard protocol decreased diagnostic accuracy, even with the greater number of counts achieved via the longer 120-minute examination.

PET and MR Imaging

The hybrid technology of PET and MR imaging offers the possibility of combining MR imaging's excellent soft tissue contrast with PET's functional imaging within a single examination. The MR imaging component of the examination may also include multiparametric techniques such as DWI (as described) or other techniques such as quantitative kinetic enhancement analysis and MR spectroscopy; multiple bioimaging markers may, therefore, be analyzed simultaneously to aid in lesion characterization. PET/MR may be performed sequentially or simultaneously with MR imaging–compatible solid-state PET detectors offering MR and PET imaging in 1 device.[51] Currently, the majority of PET/MR studies evaluate the efficacy of the radiotracer 18F-FDG; however, there is increasing interest in other radiotracers, such as 18F-labeled sodium fluoride, which may increase detection of osseous metastases.

PET and MR imaging and the evaluation of breast lesions

DCE MR imaging has a high sensitivity for detecting breast lesions; the addition of PET alone to the examination has not been shown to improve the sensitivity for detecting breast cancer achieved with MR imaging alone.[52–54] However, the use of PET in conjunction with multiparametric MR imaging capabilities has promise for improved diagnostic accuracy.[55] Pinker and colleagues[55] evaluated 76 women with either Breast Imaging Reporting and Data Systems (BI-RADS) 0 or BI-RADS 4 or 5 findings with PET-MR imaging of the breast (PET and multiparametric MR imaging [DCE MR imaging, DWI, and MR spectroscopy] at 3 T). They found that[19] FDG PET-MR imaging in conjunction with all multiparametric parameters yielded highest area under the receiver operator characteristic curve of 0.935 compared with other imaging combinations and that use of PET/MR imaging would have significantly reduced nonmalignant breast biopsies.

PET and MR imaging, and known disease

Local tumor staging MR imaging is more sensitive for detecting cancer within the breast than PET/CT and is better at detecting multifocal, multicentric, and contralateral disease in the context of a known malignancy,[54,56,57] although it is less specific than PET/CT. PET/CT, in contrast, has been shown to offer improved detection of axillary nodal involvement.[56,58] PET/MR imaging, therefore, may offer excellent assessment of extent of disease within the breast as well as axillary nodal spread (**Figs. 3** and **4**), although some studies have found that MR imaging and PET/MR imaging are not significantly different for nodal disease detection in terms of sensitivity or specificity.[54,56]

Distant metastatic disease PET/MR imaging may be performed as a whole body examination, which is particularly of value in evaluating metastatic disease and for oncologic staging. Historically, PET/CT has been used both to monitor treatment response and to evaluate for recurrent or metastatic disease in patients with breast cancer. However, PET/MR imaging offers the advantages of equivalent accuracy to PET/CT at a lower radiation dose than PET/CT.

Specifically, PET/MR imaging has been shown to have better sensitivity for liver and possibly osseous metastases, and can also detect brain lesions, although it is not as sensitive for pulmonary metastases.[59–61] PET/MR may also be superior to PET/CT, MR imaging, and CT alone in the evaluation of whole body staging in tumor recurrence. A prospective

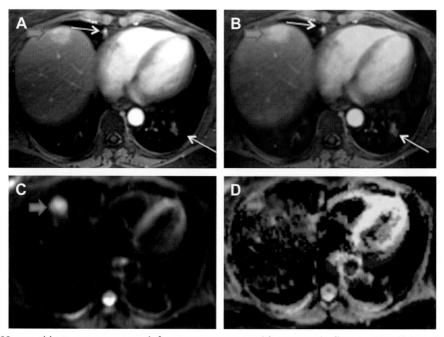

Fig. 3. A 66-year-old woman status post left mastectomy now with metastatic disease. PET/MR imaging demonstrates an enhancing hepatic metastasis in segment VIII (*block arrows*) on (*A*) T1-weighted postcontrast and (*B*) fused PET images, which is most conspicuous on (*C*) diffusion-weighted imaging and shows low signal on the associated (*D*) apparent diffusion coefficient map. In addition, lung metastases in the middle lobe and left lower lobes (*arrows*) are best seen on the T1-weighted and fused image sets (*A, B*).

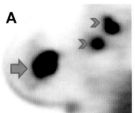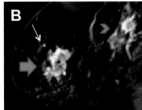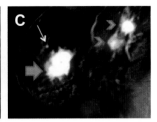

Fig. 4. A 50-year-old woman with newly diagnosed right breast cancer. (*A*) The PET image demonstrates the index breast cancer (*block arrow*) and 2 distinct metastatic axillary nodes (*chevrons*). (*B*) The postcontrast T1-weighted MR image demonstrates the spiculated index cancer (*block arrow*) in much greater morphologic detail, conglomerate axillary adenopathy (*chevron*), and a satellite lesion not seen on PET (*arrow*). (*C*) Fused PET/MR imaging images demonstrate the index cancer (*block arrow*), discrete metastatic axillary nodes (*chevrons*), and the satellite lesion (*arrow*).

study of 21 patients with suspected recurrent disease found that PET/MR imaging yielded the highest proportion of correctly categorized lesions (98.5%) compared with PET/CT (94.8%). In addition, PET/MR imaging identified all 134 lesions (100%), whereas PET/CT, MR imaging, and CT identified 97.0%, 96.2%, and 74.6% respectively.[60]

Treatment response PET/MR imaging may also be of use in predicting breast cancer response to neoadjuvant chemotherapy. MR kinetic parameters, changes in tumor diameter, change in ADC, and changes in the maximum standardized uptake value have been used to predict pathologic complete response during treatment.[62–65] PET/MR imaging has also been used to evaluate response after treatment with MR imaging showing higher specificity and PET demonstrating higher sensitivity for treatment response.[66,67]

Technical challenges PET/MR imaging is subject to a range of technical challenges. Lesion misregistration between PET and MR modalities may arise, most commonly from patient respiratory motion; a dedicated breath-hold protocol may diminish such artifact. In addition, metal artifacts can cause signal drop-out and standardized uptake value underestimation; this anomaly may be seen with breast tissue expanders.[51] Finally, work is ongoing regarding the standardization of standardized uptake value values on PET/MR imaging with active investigation of how best to optimize MR-based attenuation correction.[51]

SUMMARY

In this article, we have reviewed several new developments in breast imaging. Specifically, we have detailed the advantages of breast MR imaging at a 3 T field strength, allowing overall improvement in the SNR and image quality, as well as the special safety and artifact considerations needed at higher field strengths. We have also discussed new approaches (AB-MR imaging) with the potential to increase the overall accessibility of the MR imaging examination by rendering it a less expensive and faster screening tool. Other MR imaging developments such as DWI continue to offer the potential for increased specificity with a range of clinical applications, including neoadjuvant chemotherapy treatment monitoring. Molecular imaging technology (PEM and Tc-99 MIBI) may enable increased cancer sensitivity across all breast densities. And PET/MR imaging offers the potential of combining both functional and anatomic imaging not only directed to the breast, but also to the rest of the body in breast cancer staging. Although more studies need to be performed, many of these techniques—from AB-MR imaging to DWI to the molecular imaging modalities—offer not only better detection and characterization of breast lesions, but also, ultimately, the potential for improved identification of biologically significant disease.

ACKNOWLEDGMENTS

The authors gratefully acknowledge the help of Amy Melsaether, MD, in obtaining the MR imaging and PET images for this article.

REFERENCES

1. Saslow D, Boetes C, Burke W, et al. American Cancer Society guidelines for breast screening with MRI as an adjunct to mammography. CA Cancer J Clin 2007;57(2):75–89.
2. Zhang L, Tang M, Min Z, et al. Accuracy of combined dynamic contrast-enhanced magnetic resonance imaging and diffusion-weighted imaging for breast cancer detection: a meta-analysis. Acta Radiol 2016;57(6):651–60.
3. Glockner JF, Hu HH, Stanley DW, et al. Parallel MR imaging: a user's guide. Radiographics 2005;25(5): 1279–97.

4. Hyslop WB, Balci NC, Semelka RC. Future horizons in MR imaging. Magn Reson Imaging Clin N Am 2005;13(2):211–24.

5. van den Brink JS, Watanabe Y, Kuhl CK, et al. Implications of SENSE MR in routine clinical practice. Eur J Radiol 2003;46(1):3–27.

6. Pinker K, Grabner G, Bogner W, et al. A combined high temporal and high spatial resolution 3 Tesla MR imaging protocol for the assessment of breast lesions: initial results. Invest Radiol 2009;44(9):553–8.

7. Pinker-Domenig K, Bogner W, Gruber S, et al. High resolution MRI of the breast at 3 T: which BI-RADS(R) descriptors are most strongly associated with the diagnosis of breast cancer? Eur Radiol 2012;22(2):322–30.

8. Rahbar H, Parsian S, Lam DL, et al. Can MRI biomarkers at 3 T identify low-risk ductal carcinoma in situ? Clin Imaging 2016;40(1):125–9.

9. Djilas-Ivanovic DD, Prvulovic NP, Bogdanovic-Stojanovic DD, et al. Breast MRI: intraindividual comparative study at 1.5 and 3.0T; initial experience. J BUON 2012;17(1):65–72.

10. Medved M, Li H, Abe H, et al. Fast bilateral breast coverage with high spectral and spatial resolution (HiSS) MRI at 3T. J Magn Reson Imaging 2017;46(5):1341–8.

11. Partridge SC, Nissan N, Rahbar H, et al. Diffusion-weighted breast MRI: clinical applications and emerging techniques. J Magn Reson Imaging 2017;45(2):337–55.

12. Dorrius MD, Dijkstra H, Oudkerk M, et al. Effect of b value and pre-admission of contrast on diagnostic accuracy of 1.5-T breast DWI: a systematic review and meta-analysis. Eur Radiol 2014;24(11):2835–47.

13. Spick C, Pinker-Domenig K, Rudas M, et al. MRI-only lesions: application of diffusion-weighted imaging obviates unnecessary MR-guided breast biopsies. Eur Radiol 2014;24(6):1204–10.

14. Cheeney S, Rahbar H, Dontchos BN, et al. Apparent diffusion coefficient values may help predict which MRI-detected high-risk breast lesions will upgrade at surgical excision. J Magn Reson Imaging 2017;46(4):1028–36.

15. Santamaria G, Bargallo X, Fernandez PL, et al. Neoadjuvant systemic therapy in breast cancer: association of contrast-enhanced MR imaging findings, diffusion-weighted imaging findings, and tumor subtype with tumor response. Radiology 2016;283:160176.

16. Gu YL, Pan SM, Ren J, et al. Role of magnetic resonance imaging in detection of pathologic complete remission in breast cancer patients treated with neoadjuvant chemotherapy: a meta-analysis. Clin Breast Cancer 2017;17(4):245–55.

17. Moloney N, Sung JM, Kilbreath S, et al. Prevalence and risk factors associated with pain 21 months following surgery for breast cancer. Support Care Cancer 2016;24(11):4533–9.

18. Kim EJ, Kim SH, Kang BJ, et al. Diagnostic value of breast MRI for predicting metastatic axillary lymph nodes in breast cancer patients: diffusion-weighted MRI and conventional MRI. Magn Reson Imaging 2014;32(10):1230–6.

19. Razek AA, Lattif MA, Denewer A, et al. Assessment of axillary lymph nodes in patients with breast cancer with diffusion-weighted MR imaging in combination with routine and dynamic contrast MR imaging. Breast Cancer 2016;23(3):525–32.

20. Rahbar H, Conlin JL, Parsian S, et al. Suspicious axillary lymph nodes identified on clinical breast MRI in patients newly diagnosed with breast cancer: can quantitative features improve discrimination of malignant from benign? Acad Radiol 2015;22(4):430–8.

21. Giess CS, Poole PS, Chikarmane SA, et al. Screening breast MRI in patients previously treated for breast cancer: diagnostic yield for cancer and abnormal interpretation rate. Acad Radiol 2015;22(11):1331–7.

22. Port ER, Park A, Borgen PI, et al. Results of MRI screening for breast cancer in high-risk patients with LCIS and atypical hyperplasia. Ann Surg Oncol 2007;14(3):1051–7.

23. Kuhl CK, Strobel K, Bieling H, et al. Supplemental breast MR imaging screening of women with average risk of breast cancer. Radiology 2017;283(2):361–70.

24. Kuhl CK, Schrading S, Strobel K, et al. Abbreviated breast magnetic resonance imaging (MRI): first postcontrast subtracted images and maximum-intensity projection-a novel approach to breast cancer screening with MRI. J Clin Oncol 2014;32(22):2304–10.

25. Mango VL, Morris EA, David Dershaw D, et al. Abbreviated protocol for breast MRI: are multiple sequences needed for cancer detection? Eur J Radiol 2015;84(1):65–70.

26. Grimm LJ, Soo MS, Yoon S, et al. Abbreviated screening protocol for breast MRI: a feasibility study. Acad Radiol 2015;22(9):1157–62.

27. Heacock L, Melsaether AN, Heller SL, et al. Evaluation of a known breast cancer using an abbreviated breast MRI protocol: correlation of imaging characteristics and pathology with lesion detection and conspicuity. Eur J Radiol 2016;85(4):815–23.

28. Harvey SC, Di Carlo PA, Lee B, et al. An abbreviated protocol for high-risk screening breast MRI saves time and resources. J Am Coll Radiol 2016;13(11S):R74–80.

29. Moschetta M, Telegrafo M, Rella L, et al. Abbreviated combined MR protocol: a new faster strategy for characterizing breast lesions. Clin Breast Cancer 2016;16(3):207–11.

30. Bickelhaupt S, Laun FB, Tesdorff J, et al. Fast and noninvasive characterization of suspicious lesions detected at breast cancer X-ray screening: capability of diffusion-weighted MR imaging with MIPs. Radiology 2016;278(3):689–97.

31. McDonald ES, Hammersley JA, Chou SH, et al. Performance of DWI as a rapid unenhanced technique for detecting mammographically occult breast cancer in elevated-risk women with dense breasts. AJR Am J Roentgenol 2016;207(1):205–16.

32. Machida Y, Shimauchi A, Kanemaki Y, et al. Feasibility and potential limitations of abbreviated breast MRI: an observer study using an enriched cohort. Breast Cancer 2017;24(3):411–9.

33. Chen SQ, Huang M, Shen YY, et al. Application of abbreviated protocol of magnetic resonance imaging for breast cancer screening in dense breast tissue. Acad Radiol 2017;24(3):316–20.

34. Panigrahi B, Mullen L, Falomo E, et al. An abbreviated protocol for high-risk screening breast magnetic resonance imaging: impact on performance metrics and BI-RADS assessment. Acad Radiol 2017;24(9):1132–8.

35. Sung JS, Stamler S, Brooks J, et al. Breast cancers detected at screening MR imaging and mammography in patients at high risk: method of detection reflects tumor histopathologic results. Radiology 2016; 280(3):716–22.

36. EA1141 – Comparison of abbreviated breast MRI and digital breast tomosynthesis in breast cancer screening in women with dense breasts. Available at: http://ecog-acrin.org/clinical-trials/ea1141-educational-materials. Accessed May 31, 2017.

37. Park JY, Yi SY, Park HJ, et al. Breast-specific gamma imaging: correlations with mammographic and clinicopathologic characteristics of breast cancer. AJR Am J Roentgenol 2014;203(1):223–8.

38. Rechtman LR, Lenihan MJ, Lieberman JH, et al. Breast-specific gamma imaging for the detection of breast cancer in dense versus nondense breasts. AJR Am J Roentgenol 2014;202(2):293–8.

39. Meissnitzer T, Seymer A, Keinrath P, et al. Added value of semi-quantitative breast-specific gamma imaging in the work-up of suspicious breast lesions compared to mammography, ultrasound and 3-T MRI. Br J Radiol 2015;88(1051): 20150147.

40. Brem RF, Ruda RC, Yang JL, et al. Breast-specific gamma-imaging for the detection of mammographically occult breast cancer in women at increased risk. J Nucl Med 2016;57(5):678–84.

41. Shermis RB, Wilson KD, Doyle MT, et al. Supplemental breast cancer screening with molecular breast imaging for women with dense breast tissue. AJR Am J Roentgenol 2016;207(2):450–7.

42. Kuhn KJ, Rapelyea JA, Torrente J, et al. Comparative diagnostic utility of low-dose breast-specific gamma imaging to current clinical standard. Breast J 2016;22(2):180–8.

43. Hendrick RE, Tredennick T. Benefit to radiation risk of breast-specific gamma imaging compared with mammography in screening asymptomatic women with dense breasts. Radiology 2016;281(2):583–8.

44. Berg WA. Nuclear breast imaging: clinical results and future directions. J Nucl Med 2016;57(Suppl 1):46S–52S.

45. Berg WA, Weinberg IN, Narayanan D, et al. High-resolution fluorodeoxyglucose positron emission tomography with compression ("positron emission mammography") is highly accurate in depicting primary breast cancer. Breast J 2006;12(4):309–23.

46. Narayanan D, Madsen KS, Kalinyak JE, et al. Interpretation of positron emission mammography and MRI by experienced breast imaging radiologists: performance and observer reproducibility. AJR Am J Roentgenol 2011;196(4):971–81.

47. Berg WA, Madsen KS, Schilling K, et al. Breast cancer: comparative effectiveness of positron emission mammography and MR imaging in presurgical planning for the ipsilateral breast. Radiology 2011; 258(1):59–72.

48. Berg WA, Madsen KS, Schilling K, et al. Comparative effectiveness of positron emission mammography and MRI in the contralateral breast of women with newly diagnosed breast cancer. AJR Am J Roentgenol 2012;198(1):219–32.

49. Yamamoto Y, Tasaki Y, Kuwada Y, et al. A preliminary report of breast cancer screening by positron emission mammography. Ann Nucl Med 2016;30(2):130–7.

50. MacDonald LR, Hippe DS, Bender LC, et al. Positron emission mammography image interpretation for reduced image count levels. J Nucl Med 2016; 57(3):348–54.

51. Rice SL, Friedman KP. Clinical PET-MR imaging in breast cancer and lung cancer. PET Clin 2016; 11(4):387–402.

52. Moy L, Noz ME, Maguire GQ Jr, et al. Role of fusion of prone FDG-PET and magnetic resonance imaging of the breasts in the evaluation of breast cancer. Breast J 2010;16(4):369–76.

53. Bitencourt AG, Lima EN, Chojniak R, et al. Can 18F-FDG PET improve the evaluation of suspicious breast lesions on MRI? Eur J Radiol 2014;83(8):1381–6.

54. Botsikas D, Kalovidouri A, Becker M, et al. Clinical utility of 18F-FDG-PET/MR for preoperative breast cancer staging. Eur Radiol 2016;26(7):2297–307.

55. Pinker K, Bogner W, Baltzer P, et al. Improved differentiation of benign and malignant breast tumors with multiparametric 18fluorodeoxyglucose positron emission tomography magnetic resonance imaging: a feasibility study. Clin Cancer Res 2014;20(13): 3540–9.

56. Grueneisen J, Nagarajah J, Buchbender C, et al. Positron emission tomography/magnetic resonance

imaging for local tumor staging in patients with primary breast cancer: a comparison with positron emission tomography/computed tomography and magnetic resonance imaging. Invest Radiol 2015; 50(8):505–13.

57. Uematsu T, Kasami M, Yuen S. Comparison of FDG PET and MRI for evaluating the tumor extent of breast cancer and the impact of FDG PET on the systemic staging and prognosis of patients who are candidates for breast-conserving therapy. Breast Cancer 2009;16(2):97–104.

58. Jung NY, Kim SH, Kim SH, et al. Effectiveness of breast MRI and (18)F-FDG PET/CT for the preoperative staging of invasive lobular carcinoma versus ductal carcinoma. J Breast Cancer 2015;18(1):63–72.

59. Melsaether AN, Raad RA, Pujara AC, et al. Comparison of whole-body (18)F FDG PET/MR imaging and whole-body (18)F FDG PET/CT in terms of lesion detection and radiation dose in patients with breast cancer. Radiology 2016;281(1):193–202.

60. Sawicki LM, Grueneisen J, Schaarschmidt BM, et al. Evaluation of (1)(8)F-FDG PET/MRI, (1)(8)F-FDG PET/CT, MRI, and CT in whole-body staging of recurrent breast cancer. Eur J Radiol 2016;85(2):459–65.

61. Catalano OA, Nicolai E, Rosen BR, et al. Comparison of CE-FDG-PET/CT with CE-FDG-PET/MR in the evaluation of osseous metastases in breast cancer patients. Br J Cancer 2015;112(9):1452–60.

62. Pahk K, Kim S, Choe JG. Early prediction of pathological complete response in luminal B type neoadjuvant chemotherapy-treated breast cancer patients: comparison between interim 18F-FDG PET/CT and MRI. Nucl Med Commun 2015;36(9):887–91.

63. Tateishi U, Miyake M, Nagaoka T, et al. Neoadjuvant chemotherapy in breast cancer: prediction of pathologic response with PET/CT and dynamic contrast-enhanced MR imaging–prospective assessment. Radiology 2012;263(1):53–63.

64. Pengel KE, Koolen BB, Loo CE, et al. Combined use of (1)(8)F-FDG PET/CT and MRI for response monitoring of breast cancer during neoadjuvant chemotherapy. Eur J Nucl Med Mol Imaging 2014;41(8):1515–24.

65. Lim I, Noh WC, Park J, et al. The combination of FDG PET and dynamic contrast-enhanced MRI improves the prediction of disease-free survival in patients with awdvanced breast cancer after the first cycle of neoadjuvant chemotherapy. Eur J Nucl Med Mol Imaging 2014;41(10):1852–60.

66. Liu Q, Wang C, Li P, et al. The role of (18)F-FDG PET/CT and MRI in assessing pathological complete response to neoadjuvant chemotherapy in patients with breast cancer: a systematic review and meta-analysis. Biomed Res Int 2016;2016:3746232.

67. Melsaether A, Moy L. Breast PET/MR imaging. Radiol Clin North Am 2017;55(3):579–89.

Comparison of Contrast-Enhanced Mammography and Contrast-Enhanced Breast MR Imaging

John Lewin, MD

KEYWORDS

• Mammography • Breast MR Imaging • Contrast agent • Breast cancer detection

KEY POINTS

- The sensitivity of contrast-enhanced mammography (CEM) to detection of breast cancer is equivalent to that of MR Imaging, at least in diagnostic populations.
- The specificity of CEM is generally superior to that of MR Imaging in clinical studies.
- CEM uses iodinated contrast and a mammography unit modified to perform dual-energy imaging.
- CEM allows imaging of both breasts in multiple projections.
- CEM has advantages over MR Imaging in terms of cost and convenience, but is relatively limited in its ability to image the chest wall and axilla.

INTRODUCTION

Screening mammography remains the only test for breast cancer that has been shown to reduce breast cancer mortality in randomized clinical trials. It is a rapid and low-cost test, well-suited for screening. The sensitivity of mammography for the detection of cancer in screening populations ranges from approximately 60% to more than 90% depending on breast density.[1] Contrast-enhanced breast MR Imaging, on the other hand, has a much higher sensitivity, approaching 100%.[2] The high sensitivity of MR Imaging is not because of the inherent properties of the technology, but rather contrast enhancement; noncontrast breast MR Imaging has low cancer detection capability. With the development of digital mammography, which first became clinically approved in 2000, efforts were started to develop a technique for using contrast enhancement with mammography in order to combine the benefits of increased lesion detection from contrast enhancement with the relative low cost and convenience of mammography. Those efforts resulted in the development and demonstration of contrast-enhanced mammography (CEM) using the dual energy subtraction technique. In the first clinical test of dual-energy CEM, Lewin and colleagues[3] studied 26 subjects with suspicious lesions. Thirteen of these proved to be malignant, and all 13 lesions were shown to enhance. Later studies comparing CEM with standard mammography all showed an advantage for CEM over unenhanced mammography.[4–6] Today CEM-capable devices are commercially available from multiple vendors and are approved for clinical use in most countries, including the United States. Other names for the technique, favored by various vendors, include contrast-enhanced spectral mammography (CESM) and contrast-enhanced digital mammography (CEDM).

IMAGING TECHNIQUE

CEM is performed using dual-energy subtraction to increase the visibility of the iodinated contrast agent. Dual-energy subtraction is used, because typical temporal subtraction, in which a precontrast

The author has nothing to disclose.

The Women's Imaging Center, 3773 Cherry Creek North Drive, Suite 101, Denver, CO 80209, USA

E-mail address: John.Lewin@thewomensimagingcenter.net

Magn Reson Imaging Clin N Am 26 (2018) 259–263
https://doi.org/10.1016/j.mric.2017.12.005

mask image is subtracted from a postcontrast image, would limit imaging to only the breast and view used for the precontrast mask image. Dual-energy imaging allows imaging of both breasts in multiple projections. The dual-energy image is obtained by using a weighted subtraction of 2 images, taken one right after the other, where 1 image is acquired at a high kVp, typically 45 to 49, and the other at a standard mammography kVp, typically 28 to 32. To further increase the energy separation of the 2 images, the high-energy beam is filtered with copper, whereas the low-energy beam is filtered using filtration typical of standard mammography, with molybdenum, rhodium, or silver.

IMAGING PROTOCOL

A standard low osmolar contrast agent, typically with a concentration of 300 mgI/mL to 370 mgI/mL, is administered intravenously using a power injector. The contrast volume is similar to that used for abdominal computed tomography (CT), typically 90 to 150 mL, depending on body weight. The patient is seated for the injection, which typically takes place in the mammography examination room. Approximately 2 minutes after the injection, dual-energy image pairs are acquired of each breast in standard mammography projections, and, if needed, additional projections. About 7 to 10 minutes are available for imaging after the injection before the enhancement has faded to the point it is no longer adequate for diagnosis. The protocol is timed so that the first images are taken at peak enhancement. For bilateral examinations, it is common to alternate sides so that each breast has at least one optimally enhanced view. If there is a breast of specific interest (eg, as in a case of new cancer), that breast is usually imaged first. The number of images that can be acquired depends entirely on the speed of positioning; the actual image acquisition takes only about 3 seconds. For each dual-energy image pair, a contrast-enhanced subtraction image is computed for use in interpretation (**Table 1**).

CLINICAL STUDIES COMPARING CONTRAST-ENHANCED MAMMOGRAPHY AND MR IMAGING

Three major clinical studies have been performed comparing CEM with MR Imaging in subjects with a newly diagnosed cancer (**Table 2**). These studies typically evaluate the modalities for their ability to detect the index lesion, depict its extent, and find additional, separate lesions. A European study, in which both CEM and MR Imaging were performed on 80 subjects with a newly diagnosed

Table 1
Imaging protocol

Intravenous catheter placement	Intravenous catheter placed in forearm or antecubital vein
Contrast type	90–150 mL iodinated contrast - power injected
Power injection rate	Patient is seated during contrast injection
Delay between injection and imaging	Standard mammography views –unilateral or bilateral
Mammography acquisition	For bilateral examination, alternate sides
Typical view sequence	Right MLO, left MLO, left CC, right CC[a],[b]
Typical acquisition time	5–7 min

[a] Typically performed as a bilateral examination; can be unilateral if appropriate.
[b] Any order may be used. In cases where there is a breast of greater interest, that breast is typically imaged first. Additional views, such as spot compression, can be added.

breast cancer, showed statistically equivalent performance between CEM and MR Imaging for detection of the index lesion, with the trend favoring CEM (80/80 for CEM vs 78/80 for MR Imaging). Lesion size measured by CEM was also shown to correlate better to final pathology, although both modalities underestimated lesion size.[7] In a similar study in the United States, 52 subjects with newly diagnosed cancer were studied by both CEM and MR Imaging. This study also showed equal sensitivity between CEM and MR Imaging (50/52 for each). MR Imaging found more additional malignant foci (22/25 vs 14/25) but at the cost of more false positives (13 vs 2).[8]

A Taiwanese study of a mixture of 81 malignant and 144 benign lesions used receiver operating curve (ROC) analysis to compare CEM, MR Imaging, and contrast-enhanced tomosynthesis (CET), an experimental technique in which dual-energy tomosynthesis is performed following a contrast injection. The study found no statistically significant difference among the 3 techniques in the area under the ROC curve (AUC), a measure of accuracy.[9] AUC values were 0.878 for CEM, 0.897 for MR Imaging, and 0.892 for CET. The study also included 2 noncontrast-enhanced techniques, mammography and digital breast tomosynthesis, for comparison. AUC values for these modalities were 0.740 and 0.784, respectively. Concordant with previously published results, the 2 contrast-enhanced techniques performed significantly better than the noncontrast-enhanced techniques.

Table 2
Clinical studies comparing contrast-enhanced mammography and MR Imaging

Study	# of Subjects	Primary Outcome	Result: CEM vs MR Imaging	Statistical Result
Fallenberg et al,[7] 2014	80	Sensitivity[a]	100% vs 98%	No difference
Jochelson et al,[8] 2013	52	Sensitivity[a]	96% vs 96%	No difference
Chou et al,[9] 2015	185	Accuracy (AUC)[b]	0.878 vs 0.897	No difference

[a] Defined as percentage of index cancers detected on each modality.
[b] AUC = area under the receiver operating characteristic curve.

An example of a cancer imaged by both CEM and MRI is shown in **Fig. 1**.

ADVANTAGES AND DISADVANTAGES OF CONTRAST-ENHANCED MAMMOGRAPHY VERSUS MR IMAGING

Table 3 lists some of the advantages and disadvantages of CEM compared with MR Imaging. CEM is a less expensive test because of lower equipment costs and a shorter examination time. MR Imaging has the advantage of being able to image the entire chest wall and axilla. CEM has the advantage of being able to detect ductal carcinoma in situ (DCIS) presenting as calcifications, even with no enhancement.[10] This detection is possible, because the low-energy image of the CEM study is equivalent to a standard mammogram.[11,12] Because of this ability to detect calcifications, CEM, when validated for this purpose, would have the potential to serve as a single high-risk screening examination, as opposed to the current standard of utilizing a combination of MR Imaging and mammography. A disadvantage of CEM is the absence of a method to biopsy findings seen only with contrast, as is available with MR Imaging. In practice, if a CEM finding cannot be correlated to a specific spot on unenhanced mammography or tomosynthesis, and cannot be identified by ultrasound, a contrast-enhanced

MR Imaging is performed and the lesion biopsied under MR Imaging guidance. Adding biopsy capability to CEM should be straightforward using existing upright stereotactic systems, and various systems are being developed, but no commercial system is as yet available.

Unlike mammography (including CEM) MR Imaging uses no ionizing radiation and does not require compression. On the other hand, patients with absolute contraindications to MR Imaging, such as those with pacemakers or other implanted ferromagnetic devices, or with relative contraindications, such as claustrophobia, can undergo CEM without problem. In general, patients prefer undergoing CEM to MR Imaging due to the MR Imaging's longer examination time, potential for claustrophobia, and loud noise.[13]

For both CEM and MR Imaging, the only significant risk is contrast-related. Although iodinated contrast is generally considered to be significantly more hazardous than gadolinium contrast, the reported differences in frequency of adverse events, as well as the overall frequency, are small. Comparison of the 2 types of agents is hindered, however, by a lack of large series and a wide spread in reported outcomes, as well as variability in terminology used to describe reactions. As reported in the American College of Radiology Manual on Contrast Media, v 10.2, the frequency of serious acute reactions for iodinated contrast is estimated at .04%,[14]

Table 3
Relative advantages of contrast-enhanced mammography and MR Imaging

Advantages of CEM	Advantages of MR Imaging
Lower equipment cost	Able to image chest wall and entire axilla
Shorter examination time	Less risk of acute contrast reaction
CEM examination includes a standard mammogram (able to detect calcifications)	No ionizing radiation
No claustrophobia or loud noise	No compression
No MR Imaging-specific contraindications, such as from pacemakers or implanted metal	MR Imaging-guided biopsy is available
No risk of nephrogenic systemic fibrosis or gadolinium deposition	

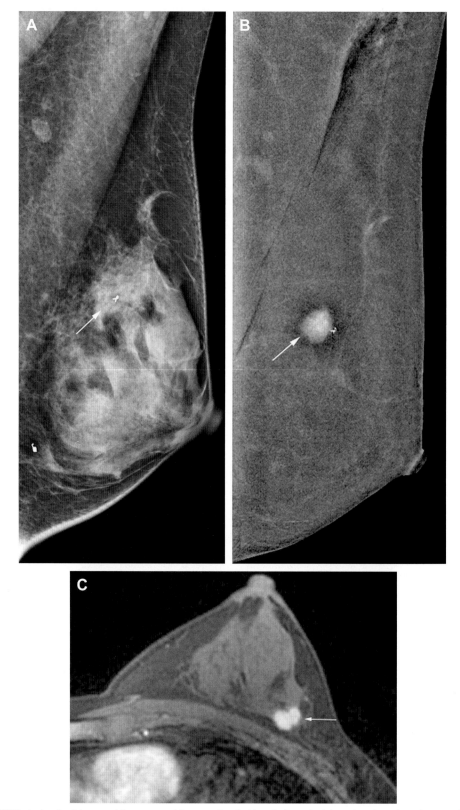

Fig. 1. CEM study of a 54-year-old woman with a previously biopsied grade 2 invasive ductal carcinoma of the left breast. (*A*) Low-energy MLO mammogram (equivalent to a standard unenhanced mammogram) shows the ribbon-shaped marker at the cancer site (*arrow*), but the cancer is not discernible. (*B*) Corresponding dual-energy subtraction image clearly depicts the cancer (*arrow*). Note that the background nonenhancing fibroglandular tissue is subtracted out. (*C*) Image from a contrast-enhanced MR Imaging performed the following day shows the lesion as an enhancing mass (*arrow*). Note the similarity of the appearance on the CEM and MR Imaging studies.

versus a rate of 0.001% to 0.01% for severe life-threatening anaphylactic reactions from gadolinium.[15] Other issues include the possible risk of nephrotoxicity from iodinated contrast and the proven but small risk of nephrogenic systemic fibrosis from gadolinium contrast. A more recent concern is the observed deposition of gadolinium in the brain from repeated administrations of the most common class of gadolinium contrast agents. Whether this deposition has any actual consequences to human health is unknown (**Fig. 1**).

POTENTIAL APPLICATIONS OF CONTRAST-ENHANCED MAMMOGRAPHY

Although studies have shown excellent performance in the diagnostic setting, CEM has not been sufficiently studied for screening; such screening studies are currently in progress. CEM is currently approved by the US Food and Drug Administration as a diagnostic test, to be used as an adjunct to standard mammography. Given the labeling, approved uses for CEM could include staging of newly diagnosed breast cancer, problem solving in cases where conventional mammography and ultrasound are inconclusive, and for evaluating treatment response in patients receiving neoadjuvant chemotherapy.

SUMMARY

CEM is in its early stages of development and clinical use. Diagnostic studies have shown similar performance to contrast-enhanced breast MR Imaging. The technique has some cost and speed advantages over MR Imaging and is better tolerated by most patients. Where CEM will fit in the armamentarium of imaging procedures available for detecting and diagnosing breast cancer remains to be seen. Most interesting will be the results of studies using CEM for screening, now in their early stages.

REFERENCES

1. Rosenberg RD, Hunt WC, Williamson MR, et al. Effects of age, breast density, ethnicity, and estrogen replacement therapy on screening mammographic sensitivity and cancer stage at diagnosis: review of 183,134 screening mammograms in Albuquerque, New Mexico. Radiology 1998;209:511–8.
2. Kuhl CK, Schrading S, Leutner CC, et al. Mammography, breast ultrasound, and magnetic resonance imaging for surveillance of women at high familial risk for breast cancer. J Clin Oncol 2005;23:8469–76.
3. Lewin JM, Isaacs PK, Vance V, et al. Dual-energy contrast-enhanced digital subtraction mammography: feasibility. Radiology 2003;229:261–8.
4. Dromain C, Thibault F, Muller S, et al. Dual-energy contrast-enhanced digital mammography: initial clinical results. Eur Radiol 2011;21(3):565–74.
5. Cheung YC, Lin YC, Wan YL, et al. Diagnostic performance of dual-energy contrast-enhanced subtracted mammography in dense breasts compared to mammography alone: interobserver blind-reading analysis. Eur Radiol 2014;24:2394–403.
6. Lobbes MB, Lalji U, Houwers J, et al. Contrast-enhanced spectral mammography in patients referred from the breast cancer screening programme. Eur Radiol 2014;24:1668–76.
7. Fallenberg EM, Dromain C, Diekmann F, et al. Contrast-enhanced spectral mammography versus MR Imaging: initial results in the detection of breast cancer and assessment of tumour size. Eur Radiol 2014;24:256–64.
8. Jochelson MS, Dershaw DD, Sung JS, et al. Bilateral contrast-enhanced dual-energy digital mammography: feasibility and comparison with conventional digital mammography and MR imaging in women with known breast carcinoma. Radiology 2013;266:743–51.
9. Chou CP, Lewin JM, Chiang CL, et al. Clinical evaluation of contrast-enhanced digital mammography and contrast-enhanced tomosynthesis–comparison to contrast-enhanced breast MR Imaging. Eur J Radiol 2015;84:2501–8.
10. Cheung YC, Juan YH, Lin YC, et al. Dual-energy contrast-enhanced spectral mammography: enhancement analysis on BI-RADS 4 non-mass microcalcifications in screened women. PLoS One 2016;11(9):e0162740.
11. Francescone MA, Jochelson MS, Dershaw DD, et al. Low energy mammogram obtained in contrast-enhanced digital mammography (CEDM) is comparable to routine full-field digital mammography (FFDM). Eur J Radiol 2014;83:1350–5.
12. Lalji UC, Jeukens CR, Houben I, et al. Evaluation of low-energy contrast-enhanced spectral mammography images by comparing them to full-field digital mammography using EUREF image quality criteria. Eur Radiol 2015;25:2813–20.
13. Hobbs MM, Taylor DB, Buzynski S, et al. Contrast-enhanced spectral mammography (CESM) and contrast enhanced MR Imaging (CEMR Imaging): Patient preferences and tolerance. J Med Imaging Radiat Oncol 2015;59:300–5.
14. Allergic-like and physiologic reactions to intravascular iodinated contrast media. In: ACR committee on drugs and contrast media. ACR manual on contrast media. V10.2. 2016. p. 23.
15. Adverse reactions to gadolinium-based contrast media. In: ACR committee on drugs and contrast media. ACR manual on contrast media. V10.2. 2016. p. 81.

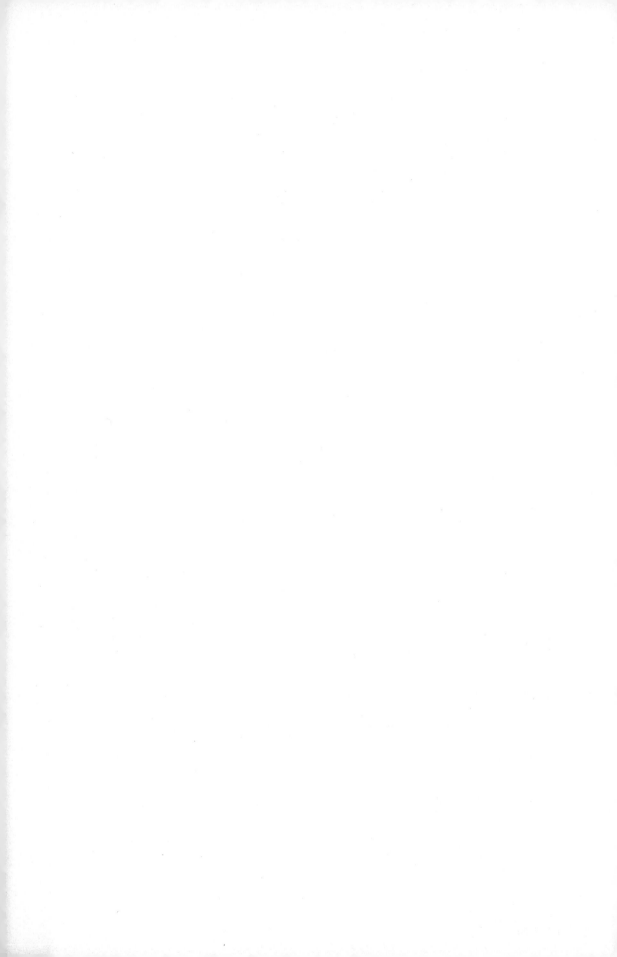

Use of Breast-Specific PET Scanners and Comparison with MR Imaging

Deepa Narayanan, MS[a],*, Wendie A. Berg, MD, PhD[b]

KEYWORDS

• Positron emission mammography • Breast PET • Breast cancer

KEY POINTS

• Positron emission mammography shows sensitivity similar to MR imaging in detecting malignant breast lesions with better specificity than MR imaging.
• Breast PET can be used in women in whom breast MR imaging is contraindicated.
• Breast imagers should interpret breast PET to assure full correlation with prior breast imaging, history, and appropriate management in conjunction with a multidisciplinary specialty team.

INTRODUCTION

Positron-emission tomography-computed tomography (PET-CT) is widely used for breast cancer staging when metastatic disease is suspected, as it provides both functional and anatomic information. Breast-specific PET has been developed to provide functional information on breast lesions with the hope of improving detection of clinically important disease and reducing false positives. Various positron-emitting radiotracers have been developed, and others are in validation, with the most widely utilized being the glucose analog 18F-2-deoxy-2-fluoro-D-glucose (FDG) with a 110-minute half-life. FDG is taken up by metabolically active cells including tumor cells, inflammatory cells, brain cells, kidney cells, and brown adipocytes, and is phosphorylated, preventing its release from the cell. Breast PET has high sensitivity for invasive breast cancer and has been validated in women with newly diagnosed breast cancer as an alternative to breast MR imaging to depict disease extent.[1,2] This article will review those data and describe preliminary results for other indications for the use of breast PET.

BREAST-SPECIFIC PET DEVICES

Whole-body PET (WBPET) and PET-CT are not optimal for evaluation of the breasts due to supine positioning and low resolution (5–6 mm), which limit detection of subcentimeter cancers.[3] Breast PET uses detectors positioned close to the breasts either similar to mammography with gentle stabilization or in the prone or semiprone position. PET requires coincidence detection of the pair of 511 KeV gamma rays emitted in opposite directions at the time of annihilation of the positron. This requirement for coincidence detection has implications near the chest wall where it may be difficult to position detectors on opposing sides without noisy background from the heart or liver.

The first commercially available breast PET system, a positron emission mammography (PEM) system from Naviscan PET Systems (currently CMR Naviscan, Carlsbad, California), now modified as the PEM Flex Solo II (**Figs. 1 and 2**), uses limited angle tomography. Patients are seated upright, and the breast is gently stabilized between clear compression paddles with

Disclosures: The authors have nothing to disclose.
[a] SBIR Development Center, National Cancer Institute, 9609 Medical Center Drive, Rockville, MD 20850, USA;
[b] Department of Radiology, University of Pittsburgh School of Medicine, Magee-Womens Hospital of UPMC, 300 Halket Street, Pittsburgh, PA 15213, USA
* Corresponding author.
E-mail address: narayanand@mail.nih.gov

Magn Reson Imaging Clin N Am 26 (2018) 265–272
https://doi.org/10.1016/j.mric.2017.12.006
1064-9689/18/Published by Elsevier Inc.

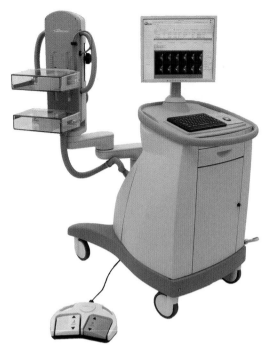

Fig. 1. CMR Naviscan's PEM Flex Solo II PEM scanner. (Photo *courtesy of* CMR Naviscan Corporation, Carlsbad, CA.)

positioning as for mammography. There are 2 opposing PET detectors that move in a linear manner within the compression paddles to scan the breast for approximately 10 minutes per image. The PEM Flex Solo II is the most widely used breast PET system to date and has been installed in over 50 sites across the United States, Latin America, and Asia. Importantly, direct PEM-guided biopsy has been developed, validated, and US Food and Drug Administration (FDA)-approved for sampling breast lesions.[4] Unlike MR imaging, specimens obtained during PEM-guided biopsy can be imaged to confirm adequate sampling and direct the pathologist's attention to the samples of interest (**Table 1**).

The MAMmography with Molecular Imaging (MAMMI) PET system from Oncovision (Valencia, Spain) is an FDA-approved true tomographic ring scanner where patients are scanned in the prone position. The breast hangs pendulous without compression within a ring of detectors that rotate around the breast. The El Mammo dedicated breast scanner (Shimadzu Corporation, Kyoto, Japan) has 2 different positioning configurations: an O-scanner where the positioning is prone, similar to MAMMI PET, and C-PEM, consisting of a C-shaped detector ring with the patient positioned semiprone leaning into the scanner. The C-shaped detector ring rotates to accommodate the arm for both right and left breast imaging. Other breast-specific PET systems are in development.[5] Although both ring and planar scanners have their own strengths and drawbacks, no differences in lesion sensitivity have been noted between them.[6]

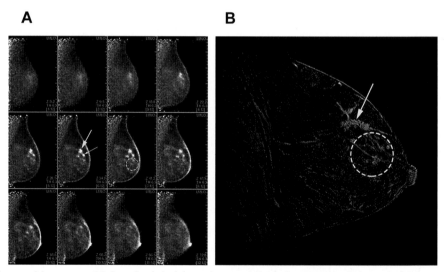

Fig. 2. 45-year-old woman with invasive lobular carcinoma. (*A*) 12-slice PEM mediolateral oblique view shows multilobulated irregular mass or group of masses spanning 3.2 cm (*straight arrows*) and scattered foci closer to the nipple (*circle*). (*B*) Sagittal T1-weighted contrast-enhanced subtraction MR image shows 3.2 cm irregular mass (*arrow*) with small enhancing foci more anteriorly (*circle*). At mastectomy, 3.0 cm of grade 1 invasive lobular carcinoma was found with lobular carcinoma in situ. More anterior foci of radiotracer uptake/MR imaging enhancement were caused by sclerosing adenosis and fibroadenomas. One axillary node was metastatic.

Table 1
Comparison of breast PET and diagnostic MR imaging

Issue	Breast PET	MR Imaging
Patient characteristic		
Weight >300 lbs, pacemaker (most), claustrophobia, allergy to gadolinium contrast	Acceptable	Contraindicated
Fasting 4–6 h	Required	N/A
Blood glucose <140 mg/dL	Required	N/A
GFR <60	Acceptable	Reduce dose of contrast if GFR 30–60; avoid if <30
Pregnancy	Contraindicated	Contraindicated
Breast implants	Acceptable	Acceptable
Examination time	40 min	40 min
Ionizing radiation	6.23 mSv[a]	None
Standardized interpretive criteria[b]	Yes	Yes
Image-guided core biopsy	Yes	Yes
Specimen imaging at time of biopsy	Yes	No
Average Reimbursement[40]	$800–$2000	$700–$2000

[a] Effective whole-body radiation dose after a single 370 MBq (10 mCi) injected dose, compared with mammography at 0.5 mSv and background radiation at 2.5 to 10 mSv per year.[12,39]
[b] Standardized interpretive criteria.[8,9]
Abbreviations: GFR, glomerular filtration rate; N/A, not applicable.

IMAGING PROTOCOL AND RADIATION EXPOSURE

In clinical studies using breast-specific PET systems, patients are injected with approximately 185 to 370 MBq (5–10 mCi) FDG after fasting for 4 to 6 hours. Blood glucose is tested prior to injection and should be in the normal range. Patients must rest quietly for 60 to 90 minutes following injection prior to commencing imaging. For PEM systems, typically both craniocaudal and mediolateral oblique views are obtained for 5 to 10 minutes of scan time per breast per view. For other systems, the scan time varies from 5 to 30 minutes per breast depending on the size of the breast.

PEM images are displayed as a 12-slice tomographic view with slice thickness equal to the compressed breast thickness divided by 12. A standardized PEM[7] interpretation lexicon that uses terminology similar to BI-RADS MR imaging[8] has been developed. Importantly, with only 2 hours' training, 36 observers showed excellent sensitivity for cancer at 96% (range 75%–100%) and specificity at 84% (range 66%–97%) in an interpretive skills task of 49 breasts including 20 (41%) cancers.[9] The same 36 observers also reviewed MR images from 32 breasts in 30 patients with sensitivity of 82% (range 45%–100%) and specificity of 67% (range 38%–91%). Interobserver agreement in description of PEM findings was moderate to substantial with kappa of 0.57 for lesion type (mass or nonmass uptake) and 0.63 for final assessment.[7]

Image quality depends on the total PEM image counts; therefore lesion detection sensitivity and diagnostic accuracy reduce with lower dose or image time.[10] Image counts can be increased by increasing either the injected activity or scan duration or both, but these cannot be boosted arbitrarily because of concerns for higher radiation exposure and/or procedure time.

Radiation dose to the patient is a significant concern for breast-specific PET imaging. A typical dose of 10 mCi (370 MBq) results in an estimated effective dose of 6.2 to 7.1 mSv, more than 10 times that associated with 2-view screen film mammography.[11] The whole-body effective dose is the sum of individual organ doses weighted by predefined tissue weighting factors. Unlike mammography, radiation exposure is to the whole body due to the systemic injection of FDG. The bladder receives the highest dose at 59 mSv, with the dose to the other organs ranging from 2.5 mSv to 8 mSv.[12] The radiation dose to the breast itself, at 2.5 mGy, is comparable to the mean glandular dose from digital mammography at 4 mGy. Considering the whole-body radiation exposure, patient preparation, and scan time, breast PET is unlikely to be used in the screening setting. Because of the high-energy emissions, shielding requirements for installing the breast PET scanner can be challenging and may require shielding of offices above and below the device.

LOCAL EXTENT OF DISEASE

There is a lack of consensus about the use of preoperative MR imaging to assess local extent and select patients for breast-conserving treatment.[13] A large prospective multicenter trial of PEM and MR imaging in 388 women with newly diagnosed biopsy-proven cancer, where breast-conserving therapy was planned, was led and reported by Berg and colleagues.[1] Of 388 index breasts with cancer, 75 (19%) ultimately were pure ductal carcinoma in situ (DCIS). For the 386 index malignancies that had surgery, with a median invasive tumor size of 1.5 cm (range 0.4–6.9), PEM depicted 357 (92.5%) versus MR imaging at 344 (89.1%, $P = .079$). Among 19 sites of biopsy-proven malignancy that were falsely negative on PEM were 11 cancers with no radiotracer uptake and 6 where the cancer could not be included in the field of view. Of 388 ipsilateral breasts, 82 (21%) had an additional 116 tumor foci not known at study entry, with a median invasive tumor size of 0.7 cm, and PEM depicted 42 (51%) with MR imaging showing 49 (60%, $P = .24$). PEM and MR imaging were complementary with 61 of 82 (74%) additional foci identified by the combination ($P<.001$ vs MR imaging alone). Importantly, review of conventional imaging showed 7 foci of malignancy (8.5% of additional foci) not seen on PEM or MR imaging, emphasizing the need for breast imaging radiologists to interpret PEM together with the patient's other breast imaging and history.

Sensitivity by tumor type was explored for the 116 malignant lesions identified after study entry.[1] DCIS was poorly detected by either PEM (23 of 56, 41% of lesions) or MR imaging (22 of 56, 39% of lesions, $P = .83$). The 59 foci of invasive cancer were less well identified using PEM at 24 of 59 (41%) sensitivity compared with MR imaging at 38 (64%, $P = .004$). Unlike studies with WBPET,[3] PEM detection of invasive lobular cancer was not worse than invasive ductal cancer. Fewer atypical hyperplasias or lobular carcinoma in situ lesions were seen on PEM compared with MR imaging.

The sensitivity of PEM and MR imaging improved with increasing tumor size ($P = .021$), as analyzed for the 40 additional foci that were greater than 90% invasive; 4 of 16 (25%) T1a lesions were seen; as were 6 of 13 (46%) T1b and 3 of 5 (60%) T1c.[1] Comparable results for MR imaging were 5 of 16 (31%) T1a, 12 of 13 (92%) T1b, and 5 of 5 (100%) T1c lesions. Eo

and colleagues[14] compared PEM tumor detection with PET-CT as a function of tumor size and showed that PEM was more sensitive for small invasive tumors (with P-value for overall sensitivity difference of 0.004); 11 of 15 (73%) T1a or T1b; 42 of 44 (95%) T1c, and 44 of 44 (100%) T2 tumors were seen on PEM compared with 9 of 15 (60%) T1a or T1b, 37 of 44 (84%) T1c, and 42 of 44 (95%) T2 tumors on PET-CT.

The multicenter PEM study showed that for the 306 breasts without additional cancer, PEM was more specific than MR imaging, with 279 (91.2%) negative on PEM compared with 264 (86.3%) on MR imaging ($P = .032$), although overall accuracy was not different. AUC of PEM was 0.72 compared with 0.76 for MR imaging ($P = .37$). Sensitivity could have been artificially reduced, and specificity could have been artificially inflated for PEM as direct PEM-guided biopsy only became available midway through the study, which would have discouraged biopsy of lesions seen only on PEM. Similar results were observed in the nonoverlapping single-center series of Schilling and colleagues[2] comparing PEM and MR imaging, and both Schilling and colleagues and a subset analysis by Kalinyak and colleagues[15] from the multicenter trial showed improved diagnostic performance of PEM compared with WBPET.

Data from the multicenter study showed that MR imaging was more accurate in surgical planning than PEM, with an accurate estimate of disease extent in 292 of 388 (75%) breasts compared with 262 of 388 (67%) for PEM. Both modalities were equally likely to overestimate the extent of disease, although PEM tended to underestimate more than MR imaging. In a recent study of 619 patients diagnosed with breast cancer, Kuhl and colleagues[16] showed that MR imaging is sensitive in depicting DCIS components associated with invasive cancer and when used with MR imaging-guided biopsy, MR imaging improved surgical treatment. In separate studies, PEM[17] and MR imaging[18,19] were found to be valuable in selecting patients for possible accelerated partial breast irradiation (APBI).

In the multicenter PEM study, 15 women were found to have contralateral cancer (median size 10 mm, range 1–22 mm) and, prospectively, only 3 (20%) were identified as suspicious by PEM compared with 14 (93%) by MR imaging ($P<.001$) with one missed on both.[20] Another 3 contralateral cancers were considered probably benign, BI-RADS 3, on PEM. On later radiologist review, blinded to results, 11 (73%) were recognized as suspicious on PEM. Lesions seen on PEM should be viewed as suspicious unless known benign by prior biopsy. A probably benign assessment,

BI-RADS 3, with short-term interval follow-up (usually in 6 months) is not appropriate for lesions seen on PEM, with 3 of 32 (9.4%) such lesions malignant in a nonoverlapping training set of cases.[7]

Visualizing tissues close to the chest wall has been a challenge for both PEM and other breast-specific PET systems. In a prospective multicenter study, 206 patients were imaged using both PET-CT and MAMMI-PET.[21] MAMMI-PET had a sensitivity of 88.9% (depicting 183 of 206 lesions), while PET-CT had a sensitivity of 91% (depicting 186 of 206 lesions, $P = .61$). Of the 23 index lesions missed by MAMMI-PET, 20 were located close to the pectoral muscle. In another single-site study,[22] Shimadzu's O-Scanner and C-scanner were evaluated and their performance compared with PET-CT and MR imaging in 69 women with 76 known or suspected breast lesions. Both O-scanner and C-scanner had similar sensitivity: 82% (62 of 76) and 83% (63 of 76) respectively. In comparison, the lesion-based sensitivity of MR imaging was 100% (76 of 76) and that of PET-CT was 92% (70 of 76). Nine lesions with the O-scanner and 6 lesions with the C-scanner were outside the field of view, thereby reducing the sensitivity of the dedicated breast PET. Like the MAMMI-PET study, all lesions that were outside the field of view were close to the chest wall and could not be imaged even with special attention to patient positioning.

AXILLA

Often it is difficult to include the axillae with breast-specific PET because of positioning similar to mammography or even on a prone table. In the prospective multicenter trial described,[1] the false-positive and false-negative rates for axillary nodal metastases were high for both PEM and MR imaging. Of 19 axillae suspicious on PEM, only 10 (53%) actually had nodal metastatic disease; of 27 axillae suspicious on MR imaging, only 13 (48%) had metastatic nodes. Of 326 axillae negative on PEM, 68 (20.9%) had metastases and of 318 negative on MR imaging, 65 (20.4%) had metastases, for overall sensitivity of 10 of 78 (13%) for PEM and 13 of 78 (17%) for MR imaging, not significantly different. Dedicated views of the axillae with the detectors in front and behind the patient's elevated arm can be obtained with PEM, but are not standard, and results with WBPET and PET-CT have not been encouraging for assessment of the axilla.[23] In a recent meta-analysis of 21 studies, MR imaging has shown to be more sensitive for diagnosing axillary lymph node metastasis compared with PET-CT with comparable specificities.[24] In a subset of patients

in the PEM multicenter trial who had PET-CT, only 8 (33%) of 24 women with nodal metastases were identified on PET-CT, and 7 of 80 (8.8%) axillae without metastatic disease were falsely suspicious.

QUANTIFICATION

Using WBPET, quantitative, and for PEM, semi-quantitative uptake of FDG have been shown to correlate with known histopathologic and immunohistochemical prognostic factors including risk of nodal metastases; greater uptake predicts response to chemotherapy.[25,26] Increasing uptake has been shown with increasing tumor grade and with triple receptor-negative tumor type.[15,25] Lower uptake has been observed in invasive lobular carcinoma.[15] Like the standardized uptake value (SUV) used in whole-body PET studies, the PEM uptake value (PUV) is a quantitative measure of the FDG uptake in the image. Although Wang and colleagues[25] have reported a high to moderate correlation between SUV and PUV in breast tissue, the PUV value differs from SUV in absolute value, because PEM images do not have corrections for attenuation or scatter. The maximum PUV for a region of interest (PUVmax) has been shown to be superior to other quantitative measures such as lesion-to-background (LTB) ratio for differentiating between benign and malignant tissue due to the simplicity and reproducibility of PUVmax.[27] Muller[28] suggested a threshold value of PUVmax greater than 1.9 as predictive of malignancy based on an analysis of 108 patients. Other studies[1,27] have found it difficult to use a discriminatory threshold for predicting malignancy, although median PUVmax for malignancies was significantly greater than that for benign lesions. In the results reported by Narayanan and colleagues,[7] the median PUVmax for benign lesions was 1.0 (standard deviation [SD], 0.4); for high-risk lesions, 1.3 (SD, 0.4); for DCIS, it was 1.1 (SD, 0.9), and for invasive malignancies with or without DCIS, it was 1.4 (SD, 0.6). $P = .001$ for differences among groups, but there was substantial overlap, with some fibroadenomas, fat necrosis, and atypical hyperplasias showing intense FDG uptake.

BACKGROUND 18F-2-DEOXY-2-FLUORO-D-GLUCOSE UPTAKE AND BREAST DENSITY

Uptake of FDG in normal breast tissue increases with visual mammographic BI-RADS breast density and decreases with patient age/postmenopausal status. An early retrospective study of 94 women with suspicious breast lesions[29] looking at a region of interest in the normal contralateral breast showed average mean (and maximum) background glandular PUV of 0.33(0.60) in fatty breasts, 0.41(0.72) in breasts with scattered fibroglandular density, 0.65(1.05) in heterogeneously dense breasts, and 0.85(1.30) in extremely dense breasts. Increasing background FDG uptake (PUVmax) was highly correlated with increasing breast density (Spearman correlation coefficient = 0.76, $P<.0001$). In a more recent study of 52 women who had both PEM and MR imaging,[30] the mean ± SD background 18F-FDG uptake on PEM was 0.25 plus or minus 0.13 in almost entirely fatty breasts (n = 5), 0.46 plus or minus 0.21 in breasts with scattered fibroglandular density (n = 12), 0.62 plus or minus 0.20 in heterogeneously dense breasts (n = 19), and 0.76 plus or minus 0.23 in extremely dense breasts (n = 16). Koo and colleagues[30] showed an inverse relationship of FDG uptake to patient age and menopausal status independent of breast density; background parenchymal enhancement on MR imaging slightly increased with increasing background FDG uptake but was not an independent predictor of FDG uptake in regression analysis. Such differences in background FDG uptake may slightly affect interpretive performance. In the multicenter study of Berg and colleagues,[1] MR imaging was more sensitive than PEM in heterogeneously dense or extremely dense breasts: 34 of 60, 57%, versus 22 of 60, 37%, P = .031. Although background parenchymal enhancement on MR imaging has been shown to predict risk of developing cancer,[31] background FDG uptake has not been studied in this regard.

RESPONSE TO PRIMARY CHEMOTHERAPY

Noritake and colleagues[32] compared the performance of PEM with that of WBPET in assessing the therapeutic response to neoadjuvant chemotherapy in 20 patients. Patients were imaged at 3 time points: before, during (interim), and after neoadjuvant chemotherapy. PEM PUVmax was highly correlated with SUVmax on WBPET (Pearson correlation coefficient r = 0.78). At the interim time point, when therapy could be changed based on imaging findings, reduction in PUVmax did not distinguish patients who ultimately had pathologic complete response (pCR) from those who did not, whereas SUVmax on WBET did. At completion of chemotherapy, further reduction in PUVmax did distinguish the 9 patients with pCR from 11 without (P = .035), although there was overlap in the groups. With increasing interest in nonsurgical approaches to women with pCR, functional imaging is of increasing potential importance to distinguish

scar from residual viable tumor. Direct comparison of PEM and MR imaging has not been performed for this indication.

OTHER APPLICATIONS

Although 1 study of 265 women, including 165 who were asymptomatic, used PEM to screen for breast cancer,[33] this will not be discussed further due to the substantial whole-body radiation exposure and patient preparation that render breast PET impractical for screening. In 1 study[34] evaluating PEM in women with suspicious calcifications going to biopsy, among 40 patients with 15 malignancies, PEM identified 14 (93.3%) cancers with 1 false-negative intermediate-grade DCIS and 1 false-positive fibroadenoma (accuracy 95%). Further study of PEM for problem solving is warranted, but may not be competitive against the much lower cost contrast-enhanced mammography. Dedicated breast PET-MR imaging systems are in early development phase at various academic research laboratories.[35,36] It is premature, however, to comment on the clinical utility. Early results with integrated whole-body PET/MR imaging have not shown superior performance in detecting breast lesions compared with MR imaging alone,[37] but technical improvements in dedicated breast PET devices may improve PET performance.

SUMMARY

Breast-specific PET imaging demonstrates high sensitivity for breast cancer and has shown promise for evaluating extent of disease in patients diagnosed with breast cancer. Although PEM and MR imaging are complementary, and the use of both improves overall performance, it is not recommended to use both because of the substantial cost and minimal added benefit in such an approach. Breast MR imaging is widely used in breast imaging clinics. Although the lack of specificity is a known disadvantage of MR imaging, there are several other factors that preclude the use of MR imaging for patients. These include contraindications to gadolinium-based contrast agents, claustrophobia, obesity, and having metal implants such as pacemakers.[38] As most of these MR imaging contraindications do not affect PEM imaging, PEM is an excellent alternative for those patients who need but cannot or will not undergo diagnostic breast MR imaging. Breast imagers should interpret breast PET to assure full correlation with prior breast imaging, history, and appropriate management in conjunction with a multidisciplinary specialty team.

REFERENCES

1. Berg WA, Madsen KS, Schilling K, et al. Breast cancer: comparative effectiveness of positron emission mammography and MR imaging in presurgical planning for the ipsilateral breast. Radiology 2011; 258(1):59–72.

2. Schilling K, Narayanan D, Kalinyak JE, et al. Positron emission mammography in breast cancer presurgical planning: comparisons with magnetic resonance imaging. Eur J Nucl Med Mol Imaging 2011;38(1): 23–36.

3. Avril N, Rose CA, Schelling M, et al. Breast imaging with positron emission tomography and fluorine-18 fluorodeoxyglucose: use and limitations. J Clin Oncol 2000;18(20):3495–502.

4. Kalinyak JE, Schilling K, Berg WA, et al. PET-guided breast biopsy. Breast J 2011;17(2):143–51.

5. Miyake KK, Nakamoto Y, Togashi K. Current status of dedicated breast PET imaging. Curr Radiol Rep 2016;4(4):16.

6. Freifelder R, Karp JS. Dedicated PET scanners for breast imaging. Phys Med Biol 1997;42(12):2463–80.

7. Narayanan D, Madsen KS, Kalinyak JE, et al. Interpretation of positron emission mammography: feature analysis and rates of malignancy. AJR Am J Roentgenol 2011;196(4):956–70.

8. Morris EA, Comstock CE, Lee CH, et al. ACR BI-RADS Magnetic Resonance Imaging. In: ACR BI-RADS Atlas. Breast Imaging Reporting and Data System. Reston (VA): American College of Radiology; 2013.

9. Narayanan D, Madsen KS, Kalinyak JE, et al. Interpretation of positron emission mammography and MRI by experienced breast imaging radiologists: performance and observer reproducibility. AJR Am J Roentgenol 2011;196(4):971–81.

10. MacDonald LR, Hippe DS, Bender LC, et al. Positron emission mammography image interpretation for reduced image count levels. J Nucl Med 2016; 57(3):348–54.

11. Hendrick RE. Radiation doses and cancer risks from breast imaging studies. Radiology 2010;257(1): 246–53.

12. Huang B, Law MW, Khong PL. Whole-body PET/CT scanning: estimation of radiation dose and cancer risk. Radiology 2009;251(1):166–74.

13. Morrow M, Waters J, Morris E. MRI for breast cancer screening, diagnosis, and treatment. Lancet 2011; 378(9805):1804–11.

14. Eo JS, Chun IK, Paeng JC, et al. Imaging sensitivity of dedicated positron emission mammography in relation to tumor size. Breast 2012;21(1):66–71.

15. Kalinyak JE, Berg WA, Schilling K, et al. Breast cancer detection using high-resolution breast PET compared to whole-body PET or PET/CT. Eur J Nucl Med Mol Imaging 2014;41(2):260–75.

16. Kuhl CK, Strobel K, Bieling H, et al. Impact of preoperative breast MR imaging and MR-guided surgery on diagnosis and surgical outcome of women with invasive breast cancer with and without DCIS Component. Radiology 2017;284(3):645–55.

17. Khanna T, El-Arousy H, Thakur N, et al. The value of positron emission mammography (PEM) in management of breast cancer. Pract Radiat Oncol 2013;3(2 Suppl 1):S24.

18. Tallet A, Rua S, Jalaguier A, et al. Impact of preoperative magnetic resonance imaging in breast cancer patients candidates for an intraoperative partial breast irradiation. Translational Cancer Research 2015;4(2):148–54.

19. Godinez J, Gombos EC, Chikarmane SA, et al. Breast MRI in the evaluation of eligibility for accelerated partial breast irradiation. AJR Am J Roentgenol 2008;191(1):272–7.

20. Berg WA, Madsen KS, Schilling K, et al. Comparative effectiveness of positron emission mammography and MRI in the contralateral breast of women with newly diagnosed breast cancer. AJR Am J Roentgenol 2012;198(1):219–32.

21. Teixeira MR, Tsarouha H, Kraggerud SM, et al. Evaluation of breast cancer polyclonality by combined chromosome banding and comparative genomic hybridization analysis. Neoplasia 2001;3(3):204–14.

22. Iima M, Nakamoto Y, Kanao S, et al. Clinical performance of 2 dedicated PET scanners for breast imaging: initial evaluation. J Nucl Med 2012;53(10): 1534–42.

23. Wahl RL, Siegel BA, Coleman RE, et al. Prospective multicenter study of axillary nodal staging by positron emission tomography in breast cancer: a report of the staging breast cancer with PET Study Group. J Clin Oncol 2004;22(2):277–85.

24. Liang X, Yu J, Wen B, et al. MRI and FDG-PET/CT based assessment of axillary lymph node metastasis in early breast cancer: a meta-analysis. Clin Radiol 2017;72(4):295–301.

25. Wang CL, MacDonald LR, Rogers JV, et al. Positron emission mammography: correlation of estrogen receptor, progesterone receptor, and human epidermal growth factor receptor 2 status and 18F-FDG. AJR Am J Roentgenol 2011;197(2): W247–55.

26. Ugurluer G, Yavuz S, Calikusu Z, et al. Correlation between 18F-FDG positron-emission tomography 18F-FDG uptake levels at diagnosis and histopathologic and immunohistochemical factors in patients with breast cancer. J Breast Health 2016;12(3):112–8.

27. Yamamoto Y, Tasaki Y, Kuwada Y, et al. Positron emission mammography (PEM): reviewing standardized semiquantitative method. Ann Nucl Med 2013;27(9):795–801.

28. Muller FH, Farahati J, Muller AG, et al. Positron emission mammography in the diagnosis of breast

cancer. Is maximum PEM uptake value a valuable threshold for malignant breast cancer detection? Nuklearmedizin 2016;55(1):15–20.

29. Berg WA, Weinberg IN, Narayanan D, et al. High-resolution fluorodeoxyglucose positron emission tomography with compression ("positron emission mammography") is highly accurate in depicting primary breast cancer. Breast J 2006;12(4):309–23.

30. Koo HR, Moon WK, Chun IK, et al. Background (1)(8)F-FDG uptake in positron emission mammography (PEM): correlation with mammographic density and background parenchymal enhancement in breast MRI. Eur J Radiol 2013;82(10):1738–42.

31. King V, Brooks JD, Bernstein JL, et al. Background parenchymal enhancement at breast MR imaging and breast cancer risk. Radiology 2011;260(1):50–60.

32. Noritake M, Narui K, Kaneta T, et al. Evaluation of the response to breast cancer neoadjuvant chemotherapy using 18F-FDG positron emission mammography compared with whole-body 18F-FDG PET: a prospective observational study. Clin Nucl Med 2017;42(3):169–75.

33. Yamamoto Y, Tasaki Y, Kuwada Y, et al. A preliminary report of breast cancer screening by positron emission mammography. Ann Nucl Med 2016;30(2):130–7.

34. Bitencourt AG, Lima EN, Macedo BR, et al. Can positron emission mammography help to identify clinically significant breast cancer in women with suspicious calcifications on mammography? Eur Radiol 2017;27(5):1893–900.

35. Ravindranath B, Junnarkar S, Purschke M, et al. Results from a simultaneous PET-MRI breast scanner. J Nucl Med 2011;52(supplement 1):432.

36. Yamamoto S, Watabe T, Watabe H, et al. Simultaneous imaging using Si-PM-based PET and MRI for development of an integrated PET/MRI system. Phys Med Biol 2012;57(2):N1–13.

37. Grueneisen J, Nagarajah J, Buchbender C, et al. Positron emission tomography/magnetic resonance imaging for local tumor staging in patients with primary breast cancer: a comparison with positron emission tomography/computed tomography and magnetic resonance imaging. Invest Radiol 2015;50(8):505–13.

38. Berg WA, Blume JD, Adams AM, et al. Reasons women at elevated risk of breast cancer refuse breast MR imaging screening: ACRIN 6666. Radiology 2010;254(1):79–87.

39. Hruska CB, O'Connor MK. Curies, and grays, and sieverts, oh my: a guide for discussing radiation dose and risk of molecular breast imaging. J Am Coll Radiol 2015;12(10):1103–5.

40. Kalles V, Zografos GC, Provatopoulou X, et al. The current status of positron emission mammography in breast cancer diagnosis. Breast Cancer 2013;20(2):123–30.

Comparison of Breast MR Imaging with Molecular Breast Imaging in Breast Cancer Screening, Diagnosis, Staging, and Treatment Response Evaluation

Gaiane M. Rauch, MD, PhD[a],*, Beatriz E. Adrada, MD[b]

KEYWORDS

- Breast imaging • Breast cancer • MBI • BSGI • Functional imaging • Breast cancer screening
- Breast cancer staging • Neoadjuvant chemotherapy response

KEY POINTS

- Breast MR imaging and molecular breast imaging (MBI) are accurate and useful supplements to screening mammography in patients at high risk for breast cancer and patients with dense breasts.
- Breast MR imaging and MBI have similar sensitivity in breast cancer diagnosis and staging. MBI has been reported to have higher specificity resulting in lower cost.
- Breast MR imaging is the most sensitive and most widely used imaging modality for evaluation of breast cancer response to neoadjuvant chemotherapy (NAC). The limited evidence available regarding use of MBI for evaluation of response to NAC shows that this technique has promise, but development of quantitative algorithms and validation with prospective studies are required.
- The advantages of breast MR imaging over MBI include absence of radiation exposure and widespread availability. The advantages of MBI over breast MR imaging include lower cost, claustrophobia-free design, absence of nephrotoxicity, and absence of limitations related to patient body weight.

INTRODUCTION

Functional imaging modalities, including MR imaging and nuclear imaging with technetium (Tc-99m) sestamibi, are gaining acceptance as adjunct modalities for breast cancer evaluation. The unique advantage of functional breast imaging over standard anatomic imaging, such as mammography and ultrasonography, is that functional imaging can reveal vascular, metabolic, and molecular changes associated with cancer before morphologic changes can be detected.

The functional imaging modality most widely used in patients with breast cancer, dynamic contrast-enhanced MR imaging, can detect angiogenesis associated with tumor growth and can also detect changes in tumor microcirculation and contrast agent uptake associated with the increased permeability of tumor blood vessels.[1] Diffusion-weighted MR imaging and its quantitative derivative, the apparent diffusion coefficient, act as a breast cancer biomarker based on the diffusivity of water, tumor cellularity, and tumor cell membrane integrity.[2]

Disclosure Statement: The authors have nothing to disclose.
[a] Department of Diagnostic Radiology, Abdominal Imaging Section, The University of Texas MD Anderson Cancer Center, 1515 Holcombe Boulevard, Unit 1473, Houston, TX 77030, USA; [b] Department of Diagnostic Radiology, Breast Imaging Section, The University of Texas MD Anderson Cancer Center, 1155 Pressler Street, Unit 1350, Houston, TX 77030-3721, USA
* Corresponding author.
E-mail address: GMRauch@mdanderson.org

Magn Reson Imaging Clin N Am 26 (2018) 273–280
https://doi.org/10.1016/j.mric.2017.12.009

mri.theclinics.com

Tc-99m sestamibi scanning is gaining acceptance as an adjunct modality for evaluation of breast cancer. Tc-99m sestamibi is a gamma-emitting radiotracer originally developed for cardiac perfusion imaging and later found to show uptake in breast tumors. The accumulation of Tc-99m sestamibi in breast tumors is due to increased angiogenesis in tumors and an increased concentration of mitochondria in cancer cells.[3] Tc-99m sestamibi is also a transport substrate for a multi-drug-resistance–associated glycoprotein, P-glycoprotein, which is overexpressed in the cell membranes of chemoresistant cancers. Thus, Tc-99m sestamibi scanning is useful in predicting sensitivity to chemotherapy.[4] Initial breast imaging with Tc-99m sestamibi, referred to as scintimammography, was performed with whole-body gamma cameras that had poor spatial resolution and were unable to reliably detect lesions smaller than 1 cm, limiting its widespread clinical use. Recent development of dedicated breast nuclear imaging devices with significantly improved resolution and sensitivity has led to increased interest in functional nuclear breast imaging with Tc-99m sestamibi.[5] These dedicated devices are usually referred to as molecular breast imaging (MBI) systems.

Breast MR imaging and MBI are used as adjunct imaging for breast cancer screening in women at high risk for breast cancer and women with dense breasts, for detecting mammographically occult breast lesions, for detecting additional ipsilateral and contralateral sites of disease during presurgical evaluation, and for predicting response to neoadjuvant therapy.

Breast MR imaging and MBI are functional adjunct imaging modalities useful for

- Detecting mammographically occult breast lesions
- Screening of high-risk women and women with dense breast tissue
- Detecting additional ipsilateral and contralateral sites of disease during presurgical evaluation
- Predicting response to neoadjuvant chemotherapy.

This article reviews clinical applications of breast MR imaging and MBI in breast cancer screening, diagnosis, staging, and treatment response evaluation; discusses the differences and similarities between breast MR imaging and MBI; and discusses the advantages and disadvantages of these 2 functional imaging techniques.

MOLECULAR BREAST IMAGING SYSTEMS

Currently, 2 major types of dedicated breast gamma imaging systems are available: single-headed scintillation detector (Sodium Iodide or Cesium Iodide) systems, commonly referred to as breast-specific gamma imaging (BSGI) (Dilon 6800, Dilon Technologies); and dual-headed direct-conversion semiconductor detector (cadmium zinc telluride) systems, commonly referred to as MBI (Discovery NM750b, GE Healthcare; LumaGem 3200s, Gamma Medica). In recent years, use of the collective term MBI to describe all dedicated breast gamma imaging systems has gained acceptance, and they are referred to as such in this article.[5] Both types of systems use standard mammographic views (craniocaudal and mediolateral oblique). The breast is positioned between a paddle and the detector for BSGI and between 2 detectors for MBI. Usually, imaging is started within 5 minutes after intravenous injection of Tc-99m sestamibi with a 10-minute acquisition per view (craniocaudal and mediolateral oblique) for each breast, for a total imaging time for both breasts of approximately 40 minutes.

BREAST MR IMAGING AND MOLECULAR BREAST IMAGING IN BREAST CANCER SCREENING

Mammography is currently the gold standard for breast cancer screening. However, mammography has limited sensitivity in screening patients with dense breast tissue and young women at high risk for breast cancer. Functional imaging modalities have been shown to overcome limitations of mammography screening, and breast MR imaging has become an accepted supplemental screening modality for high-risk women.[6]

The reported sensitivity of breast MR imaging for breast cancer detection in high-risk women ranges from 64% to 94%, and the reported specificity ranges are from 54% to 98%.[7] The reported incremental cancer detection rate for MR imaging varies from 8 to 31 cases per 1000 women screened.[8]

The performance of MBI as a supplement to mammography for breast cancer screening is similar to that of MR imaging. Meta-analysis of MBI as an adjunct to mammography for breast cancer detection showed a pooled sensitivity of 95% and specificity of 80%.[9] A retrospective study of supplemental MBI in 849 subjects at increased risk for breast cancer reported an incremental cancer detection rate of 16.5 cases per 1000 women screened, which was similar to rates with MR imaging.[10]

Because dense breasts are associated with reduced sensitivity of mammography in the detection of breast cancer, legislation in several states recommends addition of other imaging modalities for the screening of women with dense breast tissue. In addition to ultrasonography, breast MR imaging and MBI have been investigated as supplemental imaging modalities for dense breasts (**Fig. 1**). The American College of Radiology Imaging Network (ACRIN) 6666 trial included 612 participants with dense breasts who had breast MR imaging in addition to screening mammography. They reported a 17.6 incremental cancer detection rate per 1000 women versus 8.2 for mammography alone. However, the specificity in the detection of breast cancer was only 71% for mammography plus MR imaging versus 92% for mammography alone.[11]

In a separate investigation, the role of MBI as a supplement to mammography was studied in 936 subjects with dense breasts.[12] MBI was associated with an incremental cancer detection rate of 7.5 cases per 1000 women screened; the cancer detection rate with mammography only was 3.2 cases per 1000 women screened. The sensitivity for breast cancer detection was 27% with mammography only and 91% with the combination of mammography and MBI. The specificity in breast cancer detection was similar for MBI (93%) and mammography (91%); specificity for the combination of mammography and MBI was 85%. These findings were confirmed in a community-based study of 1696 women with dense breasts in which the reported incremental breast cancer detection rate was 7.7 cases per 1000 women screened.[13]

- Breast MR imaging and MBI are accurate and useful supplements to screening mammography in women at high risk for breast cancer and women with dense breasts, and the 2 techniques have similar sensitivities.
- MBI reportedly has slightly higher specificity than MR imaging.

Studies comparing MBI and MR imaging have demonstrated similar sensitivity for the 2 modalities but higher specificity for MBI.[14,15] A comparative analysis of 357 subjects who underwent MBI and MR imaging showed that the 2 techniques had sensitivities of 80% and 94%, respectively, and specificities of 84% and 67%, respectively.[15]

BREAST MR IMAGING AND MOLECULAR BREAST IMAGING IN BREAST CANCER DIAGNOSIS

There is increased interest in using functional imaging modalities for evaluation of subtypes of breast cancer that represent diagnostic challenge for standard anatomic imaging.

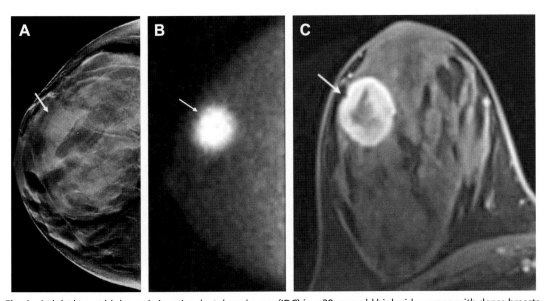

Fig. 1. A right breast high-grade invasive ductal carcinoma (IDC) in a 29-year-old high-risk woman with dense breasts. (*A*) A right craniocaudal (CC) mammogram shows extremely dense breast tissue. Known malignancy is seen as subtle (barely discernible) asymmetry (*white arrow*) in the lateral region of the right breast. (*B*) A right CC MBI shows marked (easily identified) homogenous mass uptake denoting the malignancy (*white arrow*). (*C*) A postcontrast axial T1-weighted fat-suppressed image shows the malignancy as a rim-enhancing mass (*white arrow*).

Invasive lobular carcinoma (ILC) has an infiltrative single-file pattern of invasion and is challenging to diagnose by mammography and ultrasound. Of all currently available breast imaging modalities, breast MR imaging has the highest sensitivity for ILC, ranging from 77% to 100%. ILC and invasive ductal carcinoma (IDC) have been shown to exhibit different phenotypic and pharmacokinetic features on breast MR imaging.[16] MBI shows sensitivity similar to MR imaging in the detection of ILC, and ILC and IDC have different uptake pattern and intensity on MBI.[17] A retrospective analysis of 44 ILC lesions showed that MBI had sensitivity of 89% and specificity of 79%, similar with breast MR imaging.[18] Brem and colleagues[19] compared the diagnostic performance of MBI, breast MR imaging, ultrasonography, and mammography for ILC and found that MBI had a higher sensitivity than MR imaging (93% vs 83%).

In reports on the use of MR imaging for ductal carcinoma in situ (DCIS) detection, reported sensitivity ranges from 70% to 100%, and reported accuracy ranges from 57% to 72%. A meta-analysis of 9 studies of subjects with DCIS demonstrated that the use of preoperative breast MR imaging did not improve reexcision rates and, in fact, increased mastectomy rates.[20] Studies suggest that MBI has sensitivity comparable to that of mammography and breast MR imaging for DCIS detection. The meta-analysis of MBI as an adjunct to mammography for breast cancer diagnosis

showed a pooled sensitivity in the detection of DCIS of 88%.[9] Spanu and colleagues[21] showed that the sensitivity of MBI in the detection of DCIS was 94%, equal to that of mammography (91%); the pattern of uptake correlated well with mammography with improved assessment of local disease extent.

- MR imaging is an established modality for evaluation of ILC; MBI and breast MR imaging show similar sensitivities in the detection of ILC.
- There is no conclusive evidence about the use of breast MR imaging for diagnosing DCIS, and data are insufficient to support the use of MBI for diagnosing DCIS.

BREAST MR IMAGING AND MOLECULAR BREAST IMAGING IN BREAST CANCER STAGING

Accurate assessment of disease extent is crucial for appropriate surgical management of newly diagnosed breast cancer. Excellent sensitivity of breast MR imaging in the detection of breast cancer has led to its increasing use as an adjunct modality for surgical planning. Data from a meta-analysis showed that preoperative breast MR imaging in women with a diagnosis of breast cancer detected

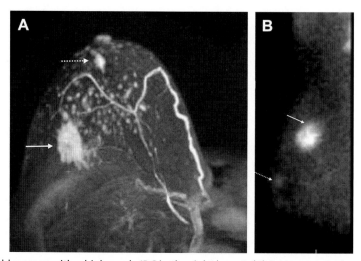

Fig. 2. A 38-year-old woman with a high-grade IDC in the right breast. (*A*) Postcontrast subtraction maximum intensity projection MR image shows known cancer as irregular mass with spiculated margins (*white arrow*). A second malignant mass is noted in the retroareolar region (*dotted arrow*). Multiple (benign) enhancing foci are present elsewhere in the breast, potentially resulting in false-positive interpretation and limiting specificity. (*B*) A mediolateral oblique MBI image shows marked mass uptake denoting index malignancy (*white arrow*) and a second malignant mass as a moderate homogeneous mass uptake (*dotted arrow*). No additional uptake is noted. MBI has been found to have similar sensitivity to MR imaging with higher specificity.

additional mammographically occult ipsilateral lesions in 16% to 20% of women and contralateral malignancies in 3% to 9% of women.[22] However, the modest specificity of breast MR imaging resulted in a high rate of false-positive findings, leading to additional biopsies and delay of treatment (**Fig. 2**). Despite extensive study, the addition of MR imaging to the presurgical workup did not show a substantial impact on observed outcomes, including reexcision, local recurrence, or survival rates. Breast MR imaging has been associated with increased rates of mastectomy instead of breast-conserving surgery.[23,24]

There are a few published retrospective studies that evaluated the use of MBI for evaluation of disease extent. In a series of 159 women with clinically suspicious breast lesions, MBI detected additional ipsilateral foci in 6% and contralateral foci in 5% of subjects.[25] In a series of 138 subjects with newly diagnosed breast cancer, MBI detected additional or more extensive malignancy in the same or contralateral breast in 10.9% of subjects.[26] Another study showed that MBI performed after mammography detected additional clinically occult ipsilateral or contralateral tumor foci, leading to a change in surgical management in 18.2% of 420 subjects with breast cancer.[27] In a study of 118 women with breast cancer for whom breast-conserving surgery was planned, 11.9% of subjects had the surgery converted to mastectomy because of additional findings on MBI.[28]

- Despite extensive study, the clinical usefulness of additional imaging for presurgical evaluation of the extent of breast cancer remains controversial.

- There is not enough evidence to demonstrate improvement of outcomes with addition of breast MR imaging, and there are no published studies on outcomes after addition of the relatively new modality of MBI.

BREAST MR IMAGING AND MOLECULAR BREAST IMAGING FOR PREDICTION OF RESPONSE TO NEOADJUVANT CHEMOTHERAPY

Neoadjuvant chemotherapy (NAC) is becoming the standard of care for patients with locally advanced breast cancer. NAC can reduce the tumor burden and thereby allow breast-conserving surgery in patients who otherwise would undergo mastectomy. The ability to predict the likelihood of pathologic complete response (pCR) early during NAC could allow for faster switching to alternate treatment options and avoid unnecessary toxicity in patients not responding to NAC.

The ACRIN 6657/I-Spy trial showed that tumor volume measured by MR imaging was the strongest predictor of pCR response early in treatment and was a strong predictor of recurrence-free survival.[29] Early prediction of pathologic response was shown in studies measuring reductions in quantitative dynamic contrast indices by dynamic contrast-enhanced MR imaging. Changes in textural features evaluated on postcontrast and T2-weighted sequences have shown promise in predicting response to NAC.[30,31] Studies evaluating diffusion-weighted MR imaging found that the apparent diffusion coefficient can reveal early intratumoral effects induced by NAC and may be an early predictor of response to NAC. A retrospective study of diffusion-weighted MR imaging in 53 subjects undergoing NAC showed significantly lower apparent diffusion coefficient values in responders than in nonresponders.[32] MR imaging is currently the most sensitive modality for evaluation of residual disease. A meta-analysis of 44 studies between 1990 and 2008 that included 2050 subjects who underwent imaging evaluation of residual disease after NAC found that MR imaging had high sensitivity (values in the various studies ranged from 83%–87%) and moderate specificity (54%–83%).[33]

MBI is a promising modality for evaluation of response to NAC. A meta-analysis of scintimammography for prediction of response to NAC included 14 studies with 503 subjects and showed sensitivity of 86% and specificity 69% in the detection of residual disease.[34] The use of newer dedicated breast imaging gamma cameras should improve the diagnostic performance of MBI; however, at present, there are few reports in the literature on their use to evaluate response to NAC. A pilot study by Mitchell and colleagues[35] evaluated the performance of MBI for early prediction of response to NAC in 19 subjects and showed that it predicted the presence of residual disease at surgery with accuracy of 89.5%, sensitivity of 92.3%, and specificity of 83.3%. In another study, the diagnostic performance of MBI and MR imaging for residual tumor detection was compared in 122 subjects, with findings on pathologic evaluation of surgical specimens used as the gold standard. The sensitivity and specificity of MBI were 74% and 72%, respectively, not very different from the sensitivity and specificity of MR imaging, which were 82% and 72%, respectively.[36]

- MR imaging is the most sensitive and the most widely used imaging modality for evaluation of response to NAC.
- The limited evidence currently available regarding use of MBI for evaluation of response to NAC suggests that it is a promising technique.

ADDITIONAL CONSIDERATIONS: BIOPSY, COST, RADIATION EXPOSURE, AVAILABILITY, AND PATIENT COMFORT

MR imaging-guided biopsy is an established and validated technique for evaluation of suspicious lesions detected by MR imaging. Until recently, a major limitation of MBI was that the only commercially available MBI systems permitting biopsy were single-headed systems; obtaining a tissue diagnosis for suspicious lesions seen on dual-headed MBI systems required additional workup with ultrasonography and/or MR imaging, thereby increasing cost. In the summer of 2016, a dual-headed biopsy device was approved by the US Food and Drug Administration, removing this limitation of MBI. However, additional studies are needed to validate the performance of biopsy with the dual-headed device.

Breast MR imaging is the most sensitive and widely available supplemental imaging modality for breast cancer evaluation; however, it has known disadvantages. The main disadvantage of MR imaging is its moderate specificity, which can lead to additional workup, unnecessary biopsies, delay of treatment, and increased cost. MBI has sensitivity similar to that of MR imaging in the evaluation of breast cancer, with better specificity and lower cost. Johnson and colleagues[37] compared the diagnostic accuracy and cost efficacy of MBI and breast MR imaging. They found that MBI had sensitivity, specificity, positive predictive value, and negative predictive value of 92%, 73%, 78%, and 90%, respectively; whereas the corresponding values for MR imaging were 89%, 54%, 67%, and 83%, respectively. Accuracy was 82% for MBI and 72% for MR imaging. The total cost of imaging was $63,750 for MBI and $253,575 for MR imaging. Major advantages of breast MR imaging over MBI include absence of radiation exposure and widespread availability. However, patients with implanted devices, severe claustrophobia, renal insufficiency, or large body habitus cannot undergo MR imaging. Intravenous gadolinium is a known cause of nephrogenic systemic fibrosis. The large number of images generated by MR imaging require long interpretation times.

Major advantages of MBI over breast MR imaging include low cost, the claustrophobia-free design of MBI systems (which allows images to be obtained with the patient in a comfortable sitting position), absence of renal toxicity, and improved specificity. Only 4 to 10 images are obtained with MBI, resulting in shorter interpretation times. The major disadvantage of MBI is the relatively high radiation dose from intravenous injection of Tc-99m sestamibi. MBI, unlike mammography, results in radiation exposure to the whole body, with greatest accumulation of radioisotope in the colon, kidneys, bladder, and gallbladder. When Tc-99m sestamibi was first used for breast imaging, the recommended and commonly used dose was 740 MBq to 1110 MBq (20–30 MCi), with an effective dose of 5.9 mSv to 9.4 mSv. However, with development of dual-headed semiconductor direct-conversion systems, an injected dose of 300 MBq (8.1 MCi) has been used in recent studies and performance has been maintained. This resulted in a decrease of the effective dose to 2.4 mSv, which is close to the 1.3-mSv effective dose from combined mammography and digital tomosynthesis.[5]

SUMMARY

Breast MR imaging and MBI have similar sensitivities in breast cancer screening, diagnosis, staging, and treatment response evaluation, with MBI showing better specificity. There is a large body of published evidence supporting the use of breast MR imaging. Given the relatively recent implementation of dual-headed direct-conversion MBI systems capable of quantitative analysis, more evidence is needed to support the use of MBI. Future research and prospective clinical trials comparing the performance of breast MR imaging and MBI and analyzing patient outcomes are necessary.

REFERENCES

1. Abramson RG, Li X, Hoyt TL, et al. Early assessment of breast cancer response to neoadjuvant chemotherapy by semi-quantitative analysis of high-temporal resolution DCE-MRI: preliminary results. Magn Reson Imaging 2013;31(9):1457–64.
2. Partridge SC, Nissan N, Rahbar H, et al. Diffusion-weighted breast MRI: clinical applications and emerging techniques. J Magn Reson Imaging 2017; 45(2):337–55.
3. Taillefer R. Clinical applications of 99mTc-sestamibi scintimammography. Semin Nucl Med 2005;35(2): 100–15.
4. Piwnica-Worms D, Chiu ML, Budding M, et al. Functional imaging of multidrug-resistant P-glycoprotein

with an organotechnetium complex. Cancer Res 1993;53(5):977–84.

5. Hruska CB, O'Connor MK. Nuclear imaging of the breast: translating achievements in instrumentation into clinical use. Med Phys 2013;40(5):050901.

6. Sung JS, Stamler S, Brooks J, et al. Breast cancers detected at screening MR imaging and mammography in patients at high risk: method of detection reflects tumor histopathologic results. Radiology 2016;280(3):716–22.

7. Warner E. The role of magnetic resonance imaging in screening women at high risk of breast cancer. Top Magn Reson Imaging 2008;19(3):163–9.

8. Lehman CD. Role of MRI in screening women at high risk for breast cancer. J Magn Reson Imaging 2006;24(5):964–70.

9. Sun Y, Wei W, Yang HW, et al. Clinical usefulness of breast-specific gamma imaging as an adjunct modality to mammography for diagnosis of breast cancer: a systemic review and meta-analysis. Eur J Nucl Med Mol Imaging 2013;40(3):450–63.

10. Brem RF, Ruda RC, Yang JL, et al. Breast-specific gamma-imaging for the detection of mammographically occult breast cancer in women at increased risk. J Nucl Med 2016;57(5):678–84.

11. Berg WA, Zhang Z, Lehrer D, et al. Detection of breast cancer with addition of annual screening ultrasound or a single screening MRI to mammography in women with elevated breast cancer risk. JAMA 2012;307(13):1394–404.

12. Rhodes DJ, Hruska CB, Phillips SW, et al. Dedicated dual-head gamma imaging for breast cancer screening in women with mammographically dense breasts. Radiology 2011;258(1):106–18.

13. Shermis RB, Wilson KD, Doyle MT, et al. Supplemental breast cancer screening with molecular breast imaging for women with dense breast tissue. AJR Am J Roentgenol 2016;207(2):450–7.

14. Brem RF, Petrovitch I, Rapelyea JA, et al. Breast-specific gamma imaging with 99mTc-sestamibi and magnetic resonance imaging in the diagnosis of breast cancer–a comparative study. Breast J 2007; 13(5):465–9.

15. Yu X, Hu G, Zhang Z, et al. Retrospective and comparative analysis of (99m)Tc-sestamibi breast specific gamma imaging versus mammography, ultrasound, and magnetic resonance imaging for the detection of breast cancer in Chinese women. BMC Cancer 2016;16:450.

16. Mann RM. The effectiveness of MR imaging in the assessment of invasive lobular carcinoma of the breast. Magn Reson Imaging Clin N Am 2010; 18(2):259–76, ix.

17. Conners AL, Jones KN, Hruska CB, et al. Direct-conversion molecular breast imaging of invasive breast cancer: imaging features, extent of invasive disease, and comparison between invasive ductal and lobular histology. AJR Am J Roentgenol 2015; 205(3):W374–81.

18. Kelley KA, Crawford JD, Thomas K, et al. A comparison of breast-specific gamma imaging of invasive lobular carcinomas and ductal carcinomas. JAMA Surg 2015;150(8):816–8.

19. Brem RF, Ioffe M, Rapelyea JA, et al. Invasive lobular carcinoma: detection with mammography, sonography, MRI, and breast-specific gamma imaging. AJR Am J Roentgenol 2009;192(2):379–83.

20. Fancellu A, Turner RM, Dixon JM, et al. Meta-analysis of the effect of preoperative breast MRI on the surgical management of ductal carcinoma in situ. Br J Surg 2015;102(8):883–93.

21. Spanu A, Sanna D, Chessa F, et al. Breast scintigraphy with breast-specific gamma-camera in the detection of ductal carcinoma in situ: a correlation with mammography and histologic subtype. J Nucl Med 2012;53(10):1528–33.

22. Plana MN, Carreira C, Muriel A, et al. Magnetic resonance imaging in the preoperative assessment of patients with primary breast cancer: systematic review of diagnostic accuracy and meta-analysis. Eur Radiol 2012;22(1):26–38.

23. Houssami N, Turner R, Morrow M. Preoperative magnetic resonance imaging in breast cancer: meta-analysis of surgical outcomes. Ann Surg 2013;257(2):249–55.

24. Vapiwala N, Hwang WT, Kushner CJ, et al. No impact of breast magnetic resonance imaging on 15-year outcomes in patients with ductal carcinoma in situ or early-stage invasive breast cancer managed with breast conservation therapy. Cancer 2017;123(8):1324–32.

25. Brem RF, Shahan C, Rapleyea JA, et al. Detection of occult foci of breast cancer using breast-specific gamma imaging in women with one mammographic or clinically suspicious breast lesion. Acad Radiol 2010;17(6):735–43.

26. Zhou M, Johnson N, Gruner S, et al. Clinical utility of breast-specific gamma imaging for evaluating disease extent in the newly diagnosed breast cancer patient. Am J Surg 2009;197(2): 159–63.

27. Spanu A, Sanna D, Chessa F, et al. The clinical impact of breast scintigraphy acquired with a breast specific gamma-camera (BSGC) in the diagnosis of breast cancer: incremental value versus mammography. Int J Oncol 2012;41(2):483–9.

28. Edwards C, Williams S, McSwain AP, et al. Breast-specific gamma imaging influences surgical management in patients with breast cancer. Breast J 2013;19(5):512–9.

29. Hylton NM, Gatsonis CA, Rosen MA, et al. Neo-adjuvant chemotherapy for breast cancer: functional tumor volume by MR imaging predicts recurrence-free survival-results from the ACRIN

6657/CALGB 150007 I-spy 1 trial. Radiology 2016;279(1):44–55.

30. Waugh SA, Purdie CA, Jordan LB, et al. Magnetic resonance imaging texture analysis classification of primary breast cancer. Eur Radiol 2016;26(2):322–30.

31. Wu J, Gong G, Cui Y, et al. Intratumor partitioning and texture analysis of dynamic contrast-enhanced (DCE)-MRI identifies relevant tumor subregions to predict pathological response of breast cancer to neoadjuvant chemotherapy. J Magn Reson Imaging 2016;44(5):1107–15.

32. Park SH, Moon WK, Cho N, et al. Diffusion-weighted MR imaging: pretreatment prediction of response to neoadjuvant chemotherapy in patients with breast cancer. Radiology 2010;257(1):56–63.

33. Marinovich ML, Macaskill P, Irwig L, et al. Meta-analysis of agreement between MRI and pathologic breast tumour size after neoadjuvant chemotherapy. Br J Cancer 2013;109(6):1528–36.

34. Guo C, Zhang C, Liu J, et al. Is Tc-99m sestamibi scintimammography useful in the prediction of neoadjuvant chemotherapy responses in breast cancer? A systematic review and meta-analysis. Nucl Med Commun 2016;37(7):675–88.

35. Mitchell D, Hruska CB, Boughey JC, et al. 99mTc-sestamibi using a direct conversion molecular breast imaging system to assess tumor response to neoadjuvant chemotherapy in women with locally advanced breast cancer. Clin Nucl Med 2013;38(12):949–56.

36. Lee HS, Ko BS, Ahn SH, et al. Diagnostic performance of breast-specific gamma imaging in the assessment of residual tumor after neoadjuvant chemotherapy in breast cancer patients. Breast Cancer Res Treat 2014;145(1):91–100.

37. Johnson N, Sorenson L, Bennetts L, et al. Breast-specific gamma imaging is a cost effective and efficacious imaging modality when compared with MRI. Am J Surg 2014;207(5):698–701 [discussion: 701].

How Does MR Imaging Help Care for My Breast Cancer Patient? Perspective of a Surgical Oncologist

Benjamin Raber, MD[a], Vivian J. Bea, MD[b],
Isabelle Bedrosian, MD[b],*

KEYWORDS

• MR imaging • Breast cancer • Surgical oncology • Breast imaging

KEY POINTS

- Breast MR imaging has superior ability to detect breast cancer when compared with traditional mammogram, and is better able to define the extent of breast disease when compared with mammography.
- Although this improved local staging alters surgical therapy in a substantial number of patients, there is no evidence to date that there is longer term benefit, such as reduction in local recurrence or reduction in contralateral breast cancer rates.
- The disadvantages associated with breast MR imaging include low specificity, increased cost, increased negative biopsy rate, and increased patient anxiety associated with increased biopsy rate.
- Given the lack of demonstrable benefit in improving patient outcomes by breast MR imaging, there are current clinical trials studying its use in neoadjuvant breast cancer treatment, surveillance, screening, and impact on patient outcomes.
- Routine use of breast MR imaging is recommended for detecting underlying carcinoma in Paget disease, identifying occult primary breast cancer in patients presenting with axillary disease, and in screening high-risk populations.

INTRODUCTION

In the late 1980s, it was determined that contrast-enhanced MR imaging could distinguish benign from malignant breast tissue.[1,2] Over time, the spatial and temporal resolution of MR imaging has increased, as the cost has decreased.[3,4] MR imaging is now readily available for surgeons to incorporate into their practice, thus, begging the question, is this new modality clinically useful? In its evolution, breast MR imaging has undergone multiple phases of recommendations, praises, and criticisms. This article discusses the current evidence-based consensus on where MR imaging belongs in a surgeon's arsenal, including the positive and negative implications of this technology.

Disclosure Statement: The authors have nothing to disclose.
[a] Department of Surgery, Baylor University Medical Center, 3500 Gaston Avenue, Dallas, TX 75246, USA;
[b] Department of Breast Surgical Oncology, The University of Texas MD Anderson Cancer Center, 1515 Holcombe Boulevard, Houston, TX 77030, USA
* Corresponding author.
E-mail address: ibedrosian@mdanderson.org

Magn Reson Imaging Clin N Am 26 (2018) 281–288
https://doi.org/10.1016/j.mric.2017.12.010
1064-9689/18/© 2017 Elsevier Inc. All rights reserved.

MR Imaging Sensitivity

It is clear that MR imaging is superior to mammogram (MMG) in the detection of disease. This difference has been proven with numerous studies, which are summarized in **Table 1**. Large single-center studies have found the sensitivity of MR imaging for the detection of breast cancer to be from 88% to 99%, with sensitivities uniformly approaching 99% when MR imaging is combined with MMG.[5–11] In 2004, Bluemke and colleagues[12] demonstrated that "additional lesions seen by MR imaging that are not visible on the MMG have been reported to be present in 27% to 37% of patients." Given the improved local staging afforded by MR imaging, it becomes critical for the surgeon to determine where this highly sensitive diagnostic tool finds its best clinical application. We review various clinical scenarios and detail the evidence for use of MR imaging in these contexts.

USE OF MR IMAGING IN PATIENTS WITH CANCER
Staging of the Primary Tumor

An early concept considered in the implementation of MR imaging to breast cancer management was the ability of MR imaging to better define the extent of disease. It was believed that the increased sensitivity of MR imaging in detecting malignant breast tissue, as previously demonstrated, would better guide surgeons in determining proper resection margins, improve the selection of patients for breast-conserving surgery versus mastectomy, and consequently decrease the rate of reoperation. Retrospective series have consistently reported on the change in surgical therapy from breast-conserving surgery to mastectomy as a result of MR staging of disease

extent, and a meta-analysis of 19 studies by Houssami and colleagues[45] noted that additional multifocal and/or multicentric disease identified by MR imaging resulted in a change in surgical therapy to mastectomy in one in six women.

Whether such a change in therapy results in reduced rates of reoperation was tested in the Comparative Effectiveness of MR imaging in Breast Cancer (COMICE) trial.[13] The COMICE trial, published in *Lancet* in 2010, prospectively randomized 1623 women with biopsy-proven breast cancer to undergo either preoperative MR imaging, or no further imaging after initial diagnosis using physical examination, MMG, and ultrasound. Surprisingly, the addition of preoperative MR imaging did not decrease the rate of reoperation. In fact, exactly 19% of the control arm and of the MR imaging arm required reoperation to obtain acceptable margins after the initial excision.[13] This trial only examined patients who were already determined to undergo breast-conservation therapy; therefore, we are unable to apply this outcome to the ability of MR imaging to prevent pathologically unnecessary mastectomy.

A second critical question is whether or not local control is improved by using the improved staging of breast MR imaging to resect mammographically occult areas of cancer. A large retrospective review from the University of Pennsylvania examined outcomes of women who underwent MR imaging before breast-conserving surgery versus patients who underwent breast surgery with no further imaging. Their results demonstrated no difference in the 8-year rates of local failure, no difference in 8-year overall survival, no difference in absence of distant metastases, and no difference on contralateral breast cancer occurrence.[14] The data were also striking for the low rates of local recurrence across the cohort; 3% in the MR

Table 1
Sensitivity and specificity of MR imaging versus MMG

	MMG Sn (%)	MMG Sp (%)	MR Imaging Sn (%)	MR Imaging Sp (%)	MR Imaging + MMG Sn (%)	MR Imaging + MMG Sp (%)
Boné et al,[5] 1997	89.0	72.0	92.0	72.0	99.0	55.0
Kacl et al,[6] 1998	82.0	64.0	92.0	76.0	95.0	52.0
Malur et al,[7] 2001	83.0	68.5	94.0	68.5	98.0	90.0
Kristoffersen Wiberg et al,[8] 2002	84.0	59.0	94.0	47.0	99.0	19.0
Teifke et al,[9] 2002	73.7	65.2	88.4	59.4	95.5	47.1
Drew et al,[10] 1999	87.6	86.4	99.2	91.0	—	—
Boné et al,[11] 2003	85	59	94	47	—	—

Abbreviations: Sn, sensitivity; Sp, specificity.

imaging arm and 4% in the no-MR imaging arm. These low rates of local failure, even in women who did not have preoperative breast MR imaging, underscore the important role of current multimodality care that emphasizes close pathologic evaluation to ensure margin-negative resection, adjuvant radiation, and adjuvant systemic therapy in achieving excellent local control. Although these data do not preclude that certain subsets of women (eg, patients at higher risk of local failure, younger women, women with denser breasts) may benefit from preoperative MR imaging, it does suggest that routine universal use of breast MR imaging for local staging as a means to better tailor therapy and reduce local failure is not warranted.

One particular group of women at higher risk are those with hormone receptor–negative cancers. The local failure rate in this population is noted to be several fold higher than those with hormone receptor–positive cancer.[15] These differences may be related to differences in radiation sensitivity and thus for the relatively radiation-resistant hormone receptor–negatives subtypes of breast cancer, use of preoperative breast MR imaging to detect and surgically treat occult areas of cancer may be relevant.[16] This question is currently being studied in the Alliance A11104 trial.[17]

Contralateral Breast Cancer

As a standard of care, women who are diagnosed with a new breast cancer undergo a physical examination and MMG of the contralateral breast. Using these two techniques, there is an 11.8% occurrence of imaging findings identified in the contralateral breast.[18] Of the findings deemed sufficiently suspicious to necessitate biopsy, nearly half are found to be cancers, yielding a 2.4% detection rate of synchronous contralateral breast carcinoma.[18] Despite the ability of physical examination and MMG to detect an occult contralateral malignancy in nearly 3 out of 100 women with newly diagnosed breast cancer, there remains a 30% rate of contralateral breast carcinoma detected in BRCA 1/2 mutation carriers, and 7% rate in non-BRCA 1/2 patients 10 years after the treatment of the original carcinoma.[19–22] The burden this second diagnosis places on the patient is immense, requiring additional trips to the operating room, and, potentially, additional exposure to radiation and chemotherapy.

The addition of MR imaging to physical examination and MMG for evaluation of contralateral breast disease after a new diagnosis of breast cancer has been shown to have a higher detection rate of occult contralateral carcinoma when compared with physical examination and MMG alone. Among the 969 women studied by Lehman and Schnall,[4] MR imaging diagnosed 30 contralateral breast cancers after having a negative physical examination and MMG. This gives breast MR imaging a diagnostic yield of 3.1%, and a sensitivity of 91%. The negative predictive value of breast MR imaging was found to be 99%. This high assurance is demonstrated in that the risk of an occult contralateral breast cancer 1 year after a negative MR imaging was only 0.3%. As the authors of that study pointed out, this information may drastically alter a patient's decision to undergo a prophylactic contralateral mastectomy in the setting of a negative MR imaging.[4] It remains unknown, however, whether the detection of contralateral breast cancer by MR imaging at time of diagnosis of the index cancer results in reduction in population level incidence of contralateral breast cancer over time.

Current National Comprehensive Cancer Network (NCCN) guidelines cite a class 2B recommendation (defined as "based upon lower-level evidence, there is NCCN consensus that the intervention is appropriate") for the use of MR imaging in contralateral breast screening at time of initial breast cancer diagnosis. Emphasis is placed on the use of MR imaging in patients with BRCA 1/2 mutations or strong family history because these are the women at greatest risk for a contralateral breast cancer, or patients with mammographically occult breast cancers.[23]

Occult Primary Breast Cancer

A rare but challenging problem that breast surgeons occasionally face is deciding what to do for patients with known axillary disease, but no identified primary breast tumor on physical examination or mammography. Accounting for less than 1% of all cases of breast cancer, these patients have historically been treated with mastectomy and axillary dissection, followed by systemic chemotherapy.[24–26] Following mastectomy, pathologic evaluation is able to identify a primary breast cancer in 30% to 60% of cases.[25,26] Multiple studies have compared surveillance to breast radiation to mastectomy, and there seems to be an advantage to primary surgical treatment with mastectomy.[27–30] Additionally, a survival benefit has been demonstrated in patients whose primary lesion is eventually identified.[31] As Blanchard and Farley[25] explain, this is likely caused the successful application of tailored treatments guided by the histology of the lesion.[31]

It is beneficial, therefore, to incorporate breast MR imaging into the algorithm for working up patients presenting with a confirmed axillary breast cancer metastasis but negative breast examination and MMG. Current NCCN guidelines have designated this a class 2A recommendation (defined as "based upon lower-level evidence, there is uniform NCCN consensus that intervention is appropriate").[23] Current studies evaluating the ability of MR imaging to identify the occult lesion have great variation, ranging from 25% to 85%.[24,32–34] If the lesion is identified, however, the patient is then able to undergo standard treatment, which may even include breast conservation or neoadjuvant therapy. In a prospective study of 40 women diagnosed with occult primary breast cancer, Olson and colleagues[26] demonstrated that MR imaging was able to identify a suspicious lesion in 70% of the cohort. Because the lesion was then identified, 27% of the cohort was amenable to lumpectomy with adjuvant radiation therapy. At a median follow-up of 19 months, none of the lumpectomy patients had a local recurrence.

A similar situation that also benefits from the high sensitivity of breast MR imaging is the patient with a known breast lesion and contralateral nodal metastasis with no identified contralateral breast tumor by examination or MMG. Given this scenario, the source of the axillary disease may be either the known primary, representing stage IV disease, or the ipsilateral breast, representing a second primary. If the surgeon performs a mastectomy on the contralateral side, a secondary breast lesion is identified in 33% to 75% of cases.[35] MR imaging can be applied in this situation to clear the contralateral breast, potentially avoiding an unnecessary bilateral mastectomy.

Paget Disease

The classic management of Paget disease is total mastectomy with axillary dissection. As with all forms of breast cancer, advances in imaging, local-regional therapy, and systemic therapy have enabled the surgeon to be much less invasive in the management of Paget disease. Presenting with a dry, eczematous rash of the nipple areolar complex, Paget disease is initially diagnosed after full-thickness surgical biopsy of the involved epidermis. Because Paget disease is associated with an underlying breast cancer in 80% to 90% of cases, it is important to image the breast after diagnosis to determine the location and histology of the underlying carcinoma.[36–38]

The treatment of Paget disease is then surgical excision of the nipple areolar complex and the underlying carcinoma. Breast-conservation therapy has been found to be oncologically safe in patients with Paget disease as long as the nipple areolar complex and any underlying lesions are excised.[36] It has been demonstrated that breast MR imaging has a superior sensitivity to MMG alone in detecting underlying carcinoma in patients presenting with Paget disease. With a positive predictive value of 100%, a negative predictive value of 17%, sensitivity of 54%, and specificity of 100%, MR imaging gives the best preoperative evaluation of underlying carcinoma in the setting of Paget disease of the breast.[36] In a single retrospective review of 69 patients over 11 years, MMG was found to miss an underlying carcinoma in 65% of cases; MR imaging was able to correctly identify the lesion in 57% of those initially missed.[36] It has been said that a negative MMG after presenting with Paget disease of the breast is an indication for breast-conserving therapy. However, given recent data, MR imaging is likely to be the determining test for these patients. For these reasons, the current NCCN guidelines give a class 2A recommendation to the use of breast MR imaging after diagnosis of Paget disease of the breast in the setting of a negative MMG.[23]

USE OF MR IMAGING IN PATIENTS WITHOUT CANCER

High-Risk Screening

When considering population-based medicine, the cost and technical complexity of a screening tool must be kept as low as possible, while still demonstrating an improvement in disease detection and survival. For this reason, MR imaging is not considered for use as a general screening tool for breast cancer. When it comes to high-risk populations, however, cost-benefit analysis may support the routine use of breast MR imaging. This was made evident in multiple studies that demonstrated that in high-risk populations, there was an increase in advanced-stage disease at diagnosis, increased lymph node involvement at time of diagnosis, and a low incidence of detecting carcinoma *in situ* using conventional annual screening MMG.[39–42]

A review article published in 2008 in the *Annals of Internal Medicine* performed a cohort analysis of 11 studies that compared MR imaging plus MMG annual screening in high-risk patients with MMG alone. The addition of MR imaging increased the diagnostic odds ratio from 14.7 to 45.9 in patients with heterogeneously dense breasts, and from 38.5 to 124.8 in patients with extremely dense breasts.[43] The evidence is clear and consistent that the addition of MR imaging to screening MMG in the high-risk population increases the cancer detection rate, along with diagnosis at earlier stage when survival is most likely to be impacted. However, the optimal age at which to begin screening with MR imaging, the age at which to stop screening, and the screening interval have yet to be determined by prospective randomized trials.

Theoretically, the implementation of MR imaging to high-risk screening should have a demonstrable impact on survival and potentially a cost savings; however, this has yet to be demonstrated in any large, prospective trials. Nevertheless, given the significant tumor downstaging achieved by MR imaging-based screening of high-risk populations, current American Cancer Society recommendations, using data from nonrandomized trials and observational studies, along with expert opinion, recommend the addition of annual MR imaging for high-risk patients.[44] At-risk groups currently considered for breast MR imaging screening as an adjunct to mammography are listed in **Box 1**.

DISADVANTAGES OF MR IMAGING

Although MR imaging of the breast has consistently been shown to be more sensitive than mammographic screening, it is more expensive and has a higher false-positive rate. In the meta-analysis by Houssami and colleagues,[45] 5.5% of

---

Box 1
American Cancer Society recommendations for breast MR imaging screening as an adjunct to mammography

Recommend Annual MR imaging Screening (Based on Evidence)

- BRCA mutation
- First-degree relative of BRCA mutation carrier, but untested
- Lifetime risk ~20%–25% or greater, as defined by models that are largely dependent on family history

Recommend Annual MR imaging Screening (Based on Expert Consensus Opinion)

- Radiation to chest between age 10 and 30 years
- Li-Fraumeni syndrome and first-degree relatives
- Cowden and Bannayan-Riley-Ruvalcaba syndromes and first-degree relatives

Data from Saslow D, Boetes C, Burke W, et al. American Cancer Society guidelines for breast screening with MRI as an adjunct to mammography. CA Cancer J Clin 2007;57(2):75–89.

---

patients had a change in surgery as a result of a false-positive MR imaging examination. These findings underscore the importance of biopsy confirmation before a change in surgical plan based on MR imaging findings is undertaken. In addition to concerns with increased false-positive rates, MR imaging is at least 10 times more expensive than mammography for screening currently.[46–50] The increased cost of breast MR imaging is in part caused by more expensive equipment, staffing needs, and more radiologist interpretation times.[51,52] Additionally, the increased sensitivity but lower specificity of breast MR imaging generates more imaging findings often requiring biopsies, which in turn can drive cost.[46] In addition to cost considerations, several authors have reported that preoperative MR imaging delays surgical treatment.[53–55] Although this delay likely does not affect survival, it can have a negative psychological impact on patients as they undergo biopsies thus delaying surgical treatment.[53] Finally, many of these series have also reported that preoperative breast MR imaging also increases the odds of bilateral mastectomy, and thus MR imaging may be among the reasons for the increasing trend in contralateral prophylactic mastectomy noted nationally.[56]

SUMMARY

Implementing breast MR imaging into breast cancer management is a complex issue. It is an expensive technology, requires highly skilled radiologic interpretation, and there are little data to suggest that it improves long-term outcomes. Nevertheless, it does have a place in the surgical oncologist's arsenal. Areas of consensus include use of MR imaging in patients presenting with Paget disease or with axillary metastasis and no obvious breast primary on standard imaging. For patients with cancer who are known to carry mutations that increase breast cancer risk or who have a strong family history, use of MR imaging to screen the contralateral breast can be considered. Use of MR imaging is also important as an adjunct to mammographic screening in high-risk populations with clear demonstration that this adjunct screening markedly reduces tumor size and nodal burden at diagnosis.

The more controversial implementation of breast MR imaging remains in defining extent of disease and as such guiding size of excision of the primary tumor. As a highly sensitive tool, breast MR imaging often recommends a larger excision. However, this does not seem to improve outcomes, especially when patients undergo adjuvant breast irradiation. Thus, routine use of MR imaging in local staging of breast cancer cannot be recommended, although individual circumstances may arise where the added sensitivity of MR imaging may be deemed useful for surgical planning.

Since its inception, breast MR imaging has been intensively studied with the goal of finding its optimal place in breast cancer management. Currently, there are 95 open clinical trials involving breast MR imaging on clinicaltrials.gov.[57] Among them are 37 trials examining the use of MR imaging in monitoring response to neoadjuvant therapy, 12 trials studying the effectiveness of new MR imaging technology, 32 trials evaluating breast MR imaging in breast cancer diagnosis (two of which are specifically studying the dense breast tissue population), seven concerning the role of breast MR imaging in surveillance after breast cancer treatment is completed, and six looking at less expensive or less invasive versions of breast MR imaging that could be used in screening.

The ability of breast MR imaging to help care for patients with breast cancer continues to evolve. As clinical trials and advancing technology give more insight into each individual patient's disease, it is up to the surgical oncologist to understand these changing capabilities, critique the emerging data, and determine how to best integrate the technology for the benefit of patients.

REFERENCES

1. Heywang SH, Fenzl G, Hahn D, et al. MR imaging of the breast: comparison with mammography and ultrasound. J Comput Assist Tomogr 1986;10(4): 615–20.

2. Kaiser WA, Zeitler E. MR imaging of the breast: fast imaging sequences with and without Gd-DTPA. Preliminary observations. Radiology 1989;170(3): 681–6.

3. Kuhl CK, Schild HH. Dynamic image interpretation of MRI of the breast. J Magn Reson Imaging 2000; 12(6):965–74.

4. Lehman CD, Schnall MD. Imaging in breast cancer: magnetic resonance imaging. Breast Cancer Res 2005;7(5):215.

5. Boné B, Péntek Z, Perbeck L, et al. Diagnostic accuracy of mammography and contrast-enhanced MR imaging in 238 histologically verified breast lesions. Acta Radiol 1997;38(4):489–96.

6. Kacl GM, Liu P, Debatin JF, et al. Detection of breast cancer with conventional mammography and contrast-enhanced MR imaging. Eur Radiol 1998; 8(2):194–200.

7. Malur S, Wurdinger S, Moritz A, et al. Comparison of written reports of mammography, sonography and magnetic resonance mammography for preoperative evaluation of breast lesions, with special emphasis on magnetic resonance mammography. Breast Cancer Res 2001;3(1):55.

8. Kristoffersen Wiberg M, Aspelin P, Perbeck L, et al. Value of MR imaging in clinical evaluation of breast lesions. Acta Radiol 2002;43(3):275–81.

9. Teifke A, Hlawatsch A, Beier T, et al. Undetected malignancies of the breast: dynamic contrast-enhanced MR imaging at 1.0 T 1. Radiology 2002; 224(3):881–8.

10. Drew PJ, Turnbull LW, Chatterjee S, et al. Prospective comparison of standard triple assessment and dynamic magnetic resonance imaging of the breast for the evaluation of symptomatic breast lesions. Ann Surg 1999;230(5):680.

11. Boné B, Wiberg MK, Szabó BK, et al. Comparison of 99mTc-Sestamibi scintimammography and dynamic MR imaging as adjuncts to mammography in the diagnosis of breast cancer. Acta Radiol 2003; 44(1):28–34.

12. Bluemke DA, Gatsonis CA, Chen MH, et al. Magnetic resonance imaging of the breast prior to biopsy. JAMA 2004;292(22):2735–42.

13. Turnbull L, Brown S, Harvey I, et al. Comparative effectiveness of MRI in breast cancer (COMICE) trial: a randomised controlled trial. Lancet 2010; 375(9714):563–71.

14. Solin LJ, Orel SG, Hwang WT, et al. Relationship of breast magnetic resonance imaging to outcome after breast-conservation treatment with radiation for women with early-stage invasive breast carcinoma or ductal carcinoma in situ. J Clin Oncol 2008; 26(3):386–91.

15. Nguyen PL, Taghian AG, Katz MS, et al. Breast cancer subtype approximated by estrogen receptor, progesterone receptor, and HER-2 is associated with local and distant recurrence after breast-conserving therapy. J Clin Oncol 2008;26(14): 2373–8.

16. Kyndi M, Sørensen FB, Knudsen H, et al. Estrogen receptor, progesterone receptor, HER-2, and response to postmastectomy radiotherapy in high-risk breast cancer: the Danish Breast Cancer Cooperative Group. J Clin Oncol 2008;26(9):1419–26.

17. Bedrosian I, Nelson H. The paradox of breast MRI: does finding occult disease make a difference. Bull Am Coll Surg 2012;97(10):57–9.

18. Morrow M, Schmidt R, Hassett C. Patient selection for breast conservation therapy with magnification mammography. Surgery 1995;118(4):621–6.

19. Metcalfe K, Lynch HT, Ghadirian P, et al. Contralateral breast cancer in BRCA1 and BRCA2 mutation carriers. J Clin Oncol 2004;22(12): 2328–35.

20. Carmichael AR, Bendall S, Lockerbie L, et al. The long-term outcome of synchronous bilateral breast cancer is worse than metachronous or unilateral tumours. Eur J Surg Oncol 2002;28(4):388–91.

21. Poggi MM, Danforth DN, Sciuto LC, et al. Eighteen-year results in the treatment of early breast carcinoma with mastectomy versus breast conservation therapy. Cancer 2003;98(4):697–702.

22. Samant RS, Olivotto IA, Jackson JS, et al. Diagnosis of metachronous contralateral breast cancer. Breast J 2001;7(6):405–10.

23. National Comprehensive Cancer Network. Breast Cancer (Version 2.2017). Available at: http://www.nccn.org/professionals/physician_gls/pdf/breast.pdf. Accessed May 9, 2017.

24. Stomper PC, Waddell BE, Edge SB, et al. Breast MRI in the evaluation of patients with occult primary breast carcinoma. Breast J 1999;5(4):230–4.

25. Blanchard DK, Farley DR. Retrospective study of women presenting with axillary metastases from occult breast carcinoma. World J Surg 2004;28(6):535–9.

26. Olson JA Jr, Morris EA, Van Zee KJ, et al. Magnetic resonance imaging facilitates breast conservation for occult breast cancer. Ann Surg Oncol 2000;7(6):411–5.

27. Masinghe SP, Faluyi OO, Kerr GR, et al. Breast radiotherapy for occult breast cancer with axillary nodal metastases: does it reduce the local recurrence rate and increase overall survival? Clin Oncol 2011;23(2):95–100.

28. Ellerbroek N, Holmes F, Singletary E, et al. Treatment of patients with isolated axillary nodal metastases from an occult primary carcinoma consistent with breast origin. Cancer 1990;66(7):1461–7.

29. Campana F, Fourquet A, Ashby MA, et al. Presentation of axillary lymphadenopathy without detectable breast primary (T0 Nib breast cancer): experience at Institut Curie. Radiother Oncol 1989;15(4):321–5.

30. Foroudi F, Tiver KW. Occult breast carcinoma presenting as axillary metastases. Int J Radiat Oncol Biol Phys 2000;47(1):143–7.

31. Abbruzzese JL, Abbruzzese MC, Lenzi R, et al. Analysis of a diagnostic strategy for patients with suspected tumors of unknown origin. J Clin Oncol 1995;13(8):2094–103.

32. Morris EA, Schwartz LH, Dershaw DD, et al. MR imaging of the breast in patients with occult primary breast carcinoma. Radiology 1997;205(2):437–40.

33. Tilanus-Linthorst MM, Obdeijn AI, Bontenbal M, et al. MRI in patients with axillary metastases of occult breast carcinoma. Breast Cancer Res Treat 1997;44(2):178–82.

34. Brenner RJ, Rothman BJ. Detection of primary breast cancer in women with known adenocarcinoma metastatic to the axilla: use of MRI after negative clinical and mammographic examination. J Magn Reson Imaging 1997;7(6):1153–8.

35. Huston TL, Pressman PI, Moore A, et al. The presentation of contralateral axillary lymph node metastases from breast carcinoma: a clinical management dilemma. Breast J 2007;13(2):158–64.

36. Marcus E. The management of Paget's disease of the breast. Curr Treat Options Oncol 2004;5(2):153–60.

37. Kollmorgen DR, Varanasi JS, Edge SB, et al. Paget's disease of the breast: a 33-year experience. J Am Coll Surg 1998;187(2):171–7.

38. Morrogh M, Morris EA, Liberman L, et al. MRI identifies otherwise occult disease in select patients with Paget disease of the nipple. J Am Coll Surg 2008;206(2):316–21.

39. Brekelmans CT, Seynaeve C, Bartels CC, et al. Effectiveness of breast cancer surveillance in BRCA1/2 gene mutation carriers and women with high familial risk. J Clin Oncol 2001;19(4):924–30.

40. Komenaka IK, Ditkoff BA, Joseph KA, et al. The development of interval breast malignancies in patients with BRCA mutations. Cancer 2004;100(10):2079–83.

41. Scheuer L, Kauff N, Robson M, et al. Outcome of preventive surgery and screening for breast and ovarian cancer in BRCA mutation carriers. J Clin Oncol 2002;20(5):1260–8.

42. Vasen HF, Tesfay E, Boonstra H, et al. Early detection of breast and ovarian cancer in families with BRCA mutations. Eur J Cancer 2005;41(4):549–54.

43. Warner E, Messersmith H, Causer P, et al. Systematic review: using magnetic resonance imaging to screen women at high risk for breast cancer. Ann Intern Med 2008;148(9):671–9.

44. Saslow D, Boetes C, Burke W, et al. American Cancer Society guidelines for breast screening with MRI as an adjunct to mammography. CA Cancer J Clin 2007;57(2):75–89.

45. Houssami N, Ciatto S, Macaskill P, et al. Accuracy and surgical impact of magnetic resonance imaging in breast cancer staging: systematic review and meta-analysis in detection of multifocal and multicentric cancer. J Clin Oncol 2008;26(19):3248–58.

46. Kriege M, Brekelmans CT, Boetes C, et al. Efficacy of MRI and mammography for breast-cancer screening in women with a familial or genetic predisposition. N Engl J Med 2004;351(5):427–37.

47. Leach MO, Boggis CR, Dixon AK, et al, MARIBS Study Group. Screening with magnetic resonance imaging and mammography of a UK population at high familial risk of breast cancer: a prospective multicentre cohort study (MARIBS). Lancet 2005;365(9473):1769–78.

48. Warner E, Plewes DB, Hill KA, et al. Surveillance of BRCA1 and BRCA2 mutation carriers with magnetic resonance imaging, ultrasound, mammography, and clinical breast examination. JAMA 2004;292(11):1317–25.

49. Plevritis SK, Kurian AW, Sigal BM, et al. Cost-effectiveness of screening BRCA1/2 mutation carriers

with breast magnetic resonance imaging. JAMA 2006;295(20):2374–84.

50. Trecate G, Vergnaghi D, Manoukian S, et al. MRI in the early detection of breast cancer in women with high genetic risk. Tumori 2006;92(6):517.

51. Patel BK, Gray RJ, Pockaj BA. Potential cost savings of contrast-enhanced digital mammography. AJR Am J Roentgenol 2017;208(6):W231–7.

52. Kuhl CK, Schrading S, Strobel K, et al. Abbreviated breast magnetic resonance imaging (MRI): first postcontrast subtracted images and maximum-intensity projection—a novel approach to breast cancer screening with MRI. J Clin Oncol 2014; 32(22):2304–10.

53. Bleicher RJ, Ciocca RM, Egleston BL, et al. Association of routine pretreatment magnetic resonance imaging with time to surgery, mastectomy rate, and margin status. J Am Coll Surg 2009; 209(2):180–7.

54. Barber MD, Jack W, Dixon JM. Diagnostic delay in breast cancer. Br J Surg 2004;91(1):49–53.

55. Richards MA, Westcombe AM, Love SB, et al. Influence of delay on survival in patients with breast cancer: a systematic review. Lancet 1999;353(9159): 1119–26.

56. Yao K, Stewart AK, Winchester DJ, et al. Trends in contralateral prophylactic mastectomy for unilateral cancer: a report from the National Cancer Data Base, 1998–2007. Ann Surg Oncol 2010;17(10): 2554–62.

57. Search for studies. Home - ClinicalTrials.gov. N.p., n.d. Web. 2017. Available at: https://clinicaltrials.gov/ct2/results?term=breast+MRI&recr=Open&pg=1. Accessed May 21, 2017.

How Does MR Imaging Help Care for the Breast Cancer Patient? Perspective of a Medical Oncologist

Akshara S. Raghavendra, MD, MS, Debu Tripathy, MD*

KEYWORDS

• MR imaging • Staging • Breast cancer • Neoadjuvant chemotherapy • Metastatic

KEY POINTS

• MR imaging can detect occult breast cancers and nodes that are not apparent during mammographic, ultrasound, or clinical workup, which may affect treatment outcome.
• MR imaging is often used to characterize extent of disease and monitor clinical response to neoadjuvant systemic therapy, to guide surgical planning; it holds the potential to predict pathologic response.
• MR imaging assists in early staging for treatment planning, as well as staging in (advanced) metastatic disease.

INTRODUCTION

MR imaging has demonstrated superior sensitivity for invasive and in situ cancer detection,[1–6] as well as more accurate determination of disease extent, when compared with physical examination, mammography, and ultrasound.[7,8] Hence, it is now recognized as an important adjunct imaging modality in the evaluation of patients with newly diagnosed breast cancer. The American College of Radiology guidelines for the performance of MR imaging[9] related to breast cancer imaging include evaluation of extent of disease for a known cancer, screening of high-risk patients, screening of the contralateral breast for patients with a new breast malignancy, and assessing response to neoadjuvant chemotherapy (NAC). However, its use has not clearly been linked to improved outcomes in all these situations and, therefore,

variations in practice exist. This article reviews the role of MR imaging from the perspective of a medical oncologist, including its ability to diagnose earlier stage disease, assessment of preoperative extent of disease in patients with newly diagnosed breast cancer, and monitoring of response to NAC, as well as its application in specific clinical scenarios among metastatic subpopulations.

By allowing for earlier detection, use of MR imaging may result in diagnosis at an earlier stage and fewer patients requiring systemic therapy, particularly chemotherapy. Simultaneously, staging with MR imaging may upstage patients and identify those who may need more aggressive systemic therapy. With regard to breast cancer survival, it has been proven that NAC is as effective as adjuvant (postoperative) chemotherapy in lowering recurrence and mortality; however, it

The authors have nothing to disclose.
Department of Breast Medical Oncology, Division of Cancer Medicine, The University of Texas MD Anderson Cancer Center, 1515 Holcombe Boulevard, Houston, TX 77030, USA
* Corresponding author. Department of Breast Medical Oncology, The University of Texas MD Anderson Cancer Center, 1515 Holcombe Boulevard, Unit 1354, Houston, TX 77030.
E-mail address: dtripathy@mdanderson.org

Magn Reson Imaging Clin N Am 26 (2018) 289–293
https://doi.org/10.1016/j.mric.2017.12.013
1064-9689/18/© 2017 Elsevier Inc. All rights reserved.

can also enable breast-conserving surgery and less aggressive lymph node excision.[10] The biological heterogeneity of breast cancer, however, results in variable responses to NAC. Ongoing trials are attempting to use response and MR imaging parameter changes over time to personalize therapy and accelerate drug development.[11]

Detection of Additional Disease in the Newly Diagnosed Patient with Breast Cancer

Evidence from 19 studies, reviewed in a meta-analysis by Houssami and colleagues,[12] showed MR imaging had a higher sensitivity for the detection of multifocal or multicentric breast cancer than conventional imaging. MR imaging identified additional foci in 16% of subjects (previously published individual studies reported a range of 6%–34%[13]), resulting in surgical decision change from wide local excision to mastectomy in 8.1% of women and a larger local excision in 11.3% of women.[12] Similarly, in another meta-analysis, MR imaging detected additional foci in 20% of subjects.[14] In the contralateral breast, MR imaging has been reported to detect additional synchronous cancers in 4.1% of subjects, with 65% of the cancer being invasive.[15]

Although extensive data exist regarding the use of MR imaging in detecting multifocal and multicentric disease, there is much controversy in the analysis of treatment outcomes differences as a result of MR imaging.[14] Hence, the true clinical contribution of breast MR imaging in this setting remains ambiguous and needs further studies.

Tumor Vascularity and Ductal Carcinoma In Situ in Upstaging Disease

Because breast cancers rely on neoangiogenesis and on the development of blood microvessels for their growth, increased vascularity in the whole ipsilateral breast may indicate the presence of disease.[16] During the past 10 years, several studies have evaluated the association between asymmetric increased breast vascularity (AIBV) on MR imaging and ipsilateral breast cancer.[16] Ipsilateral AIBV was associated with a more aggressive clinical, pathologic, and molecular profile.[16] This may be interpreted as the consequence of more proangiogenic signals released by highly proliferating cancers.[16] MR imaging is reliable for the analysis of whole breast vascularity. The assessment of vascular maps and of AIBV could represent an additional information for tumor characterization and treatment planning.[16] One study showed that with the use of MR imaging in patients with a preoperative diagnosis of ductal carcinoma in situ (DCIS), the rate of upstaging of DCIS to

invasive cancer was 26.7% (35 to 131), emphasizing the role of MR imaging in triaging patients who are at highest risk for occult invasive disease.[17]

Breast Cancer Subtypes

Breast cancer subtypes based on hormone and human epidermal growth factor receptor 2 (HER2) status are used for medical treatment decision. More recent classifications based on gene expression or mutational profiles are being investigated. In a trial conducted by the Translational Breast Cancer Research Consortium, MR imaging detected breast cancer with an overall accuracy of 74%, varying among molecular subtypes.[18] Dynamic contrast-enhanced (DCE)–MR imaging has the ability to depict the physiologic tissue characteristics as a whole tumor and has strong potential use in the management of breast cancer.[19]

Because of the heterogeneity of tumor in patients with triple-negative breast cancer (TNBC) and their varied response to chemotherapy, a combination of treatment planning is important in prognostication. TNBC has distinctive MR imaging features. It appears as a unifocal mass, whereas HER2-positive tumors may be seen as multiple masses at diagnosis. Therefore, MR imaging may prove more effective in depicting TNBC and HER2-positive tumor subtype.[20]

MR imaging is useful for predicting the likelihood of pathologic complete response (pCR) among tumor subtypes following NAC. In a study of 188 women using MR imaging, analysis of residual disease showed significant associations with change in the diameter of the tumor during NAC for TNBC and HER2-positive tumors.[21] Another extensive study demonstrated the utility of DCE–MR imaging by analyzing the biomarker status among NAC patients who had an increase in pCR rate by 46% in TNBC and 73% in nonluminal-positive or HER2-positive subtypes.[22] Functional imaging, such as DCE–MR imaging, promises great clinical potential in its ability to assign biologically driven therapies based on characteristics such as increased metabolism, proliferation, or vascularity. Prospective trials assessing the benefits imparted from MR imaging–driven treatment decisions will be needed; many are currently in progress.

Predicting Tumor Response

Several studies have evaluated the utility of MR imaging performed for staging breast cancer, as well as predicting clinical or pathologic tumor response, which correlated with a long-term disease-free state and overall survival.[23–31] Contrast-enhanced MR imaging is considered the most accurate imaging modality for invasive breast cancer[32,33] and is increasingly used for the evaluation of NAC response.[34] Previously published criteria considered a reduction of more than 25% of the tumor measured in the largest diameter on interim MR imaging as a satisfactory response during chemotherapy.[35] This was termed a favorable response; anything less was classified as unfavorable.[34] Although DCE–MR imaging accurately evaluates the extent of primary breast cancer,[32,33] it was shown not to be a decisive predictor of pathologic response.[21] Nevertheless, an unfavorable response on the interim MR imaging did correlate with a lower rate of pCR of the breast.[34] Analysis of these patients does suggest that a switch in chemotherapy regimen may still be effective when the initial chemotherapy is not.[34] Imaging after chemotherapy showed significantly improved performance over imaging before chemotherapy for predicting residual tumor.[19] A subgroup analysis of 216 subjects of the American College of Radiology Imaging Network (ACRIN) 6657/I-SPY 1 trial studied the effect of MR imaging in predicting the response to NAC, and the findings suggested that measuring the tumor volume on interim MR imaging was useful for predicting pathologic response, as well as for treatment planning.[36]

MR imaging response to NAC may also be used to predict recurrence-free survival (RFS) and this can help identify patients who may be candidates for more aggressive adjuvant therapy or enrollment in adjuvant trials. In a study of 58 subjects with nonmetastatic breast cancer who received NAC, changes in the tumor volume at MR imaging showed an association with RFS.[37]

Higher background parenchymal enhancement of the contralateral breast at MR imaging is significantly associated with poor RFS in patients who underwent NAC for a unilateral invasive breast cancer.[38] Several prospective studies are using MR imaging to further personalize therapy and to accelerate the development of novel agents using MR imaging response as a surrogate to long-term outcome. However, currently, there is no universally accepted standard to deviate from accepted adjuvant regimens based on changes with MR imaging alone.

Staging Metastatic Disease

The early detection and follow-up of the patient with metastatic breast cancer is important because of drastic treatment-changing paradigms.[39] Whole-body MR imaging is the preferred imaging modality for assessing metastatic spread in the marrow cavity and surrounding structures due to its high soft tissue resolution.[40] MR imaging is 95% sensitive and 90% specific for detection of bone metastasis and is especially useful in pregnant women because nonenhanced MR imaging is safer than ionizing computed tomography during pregnancy.[41]

In addition, MR imaging is the gold standard in imaging suspected cases of cord compression, demonstrating pathologic vertebral body fracture, which is considered a medical emergency. If undetected, it can result in irreversible neurologic damage. MR imaging sequences can detect abnormal focal high T2 and/or turbo-short tau inversion recovery signal.[41]

Because of is excellent soft tissue resolution, MR imaging is particularly helpful for detecting metastatic disease (which may be seen as a focal mass) affecting the brachial plexus. Accordingly, MR imaging is helpful in the differentiation between radiation-induced versus neoplastic brachial plexopathy.[42]

Diagnosis of leptomeningeal metastasis has become increasingly frequent. The diagnostic gold standard traditionally has been cytology from cerebrospinal fluid; however, MR imaging is now used routinely for diagnosis based on leptomeningeal enhancement, which, along with clinical findings, can establish the diagnosis and alter therapy. Nodular enhancement of the leptomeninges or cranial nerves is suggestive of leptomeningeal metastasis.[43]

Breast Cancer Presenting as Unknown Primary Tumor

Breast cancers presenting with axillary lymph node metastasis with an undetectable primary breast tumor by standard clinical examination and conventional imaging make up less than 1% of all breast cancers. In a previously published meta-analysis of 8 retrospective studies, MR imaging revealed the primary breast cancer in 72% of cases, with a sensitivity of 90% and a specificity of 31% (tumor size ranged from 5 mm to 16 mm).[44]

SUMMARY

MR imaging is among the most sensitive imaging modalities in routine clinical practice and highly correlative with disease and vascularity. The use of breast MR imaging for assessment of the extent of the disease in patients with newly diagnosed breast cancer remains controversial because studies have not clearly shown benefits in terms of reoperation rate, disease recurrence, or survival. Further studies addressing these questions will require time and multiinstitutional collaboration to demonstrate improvement over the already low recurrence and high survival rates in patients undergoing breast-conserving therapy. Nevertheless, there are select subpopulations that may benefit from preoperative MR imaging, and further study in defined subpopulations may indeed show that MR imaging is beneficial in specific groups to warrant certain medical interventions.

MR imaging has been shown to be valuable in assessing response to NAC. In general, given the imperfect specificity of breast MR imaging, all suspicious MR imaging findings should be correlated with biopsy results before definitive cancer therapy to ensure appropriate and optimal treatment. The integration of MR imaging into research trials testing new drugs in the neoadjuvant and advanced disease settings may accelerate discovery by providing a quicker readout of response and may allow for the testing of early regimen switching in a personalized manner.

REFERENCES

1. Bedrosian I, Mick R, Orel SG, et al. Changes in the surgical management of patients with breast carcinoma based on preoperative magnetic resonance imaging. Cancer 2003;98:468–73.
2. Lehman CD, Blume JD, Thickman D, et al. Added cancer yield of MRI in screening the contralateral breast of women recently diagnosed with breast cancer: results from the International Breast Magnetic Resonance Consortium (IBMC) trial. J Surg Oncol 2005;92:9–15.
3. Liberman L, Morris EA, Dershaw DD, et al. MR imaging of the ipsilateral breast in women with percutaneously proven breast cancer. AJR Am J Roentgenol 2003;180:901–10.
4. Orel SG, Schnall MD, Powell CM, et al. Staging of suspected breast cancer: effect of MR imaging and MR-guided biopsy. Radiology 1995;196:115–22.
5. Rieber A, Merkle E, Böhm W, et al. MRI of histologically confirmed mammary carcinoma: clinical relevance of diagnostic procedures for detection of multifocal or contralateral secondary carcinoma. J Comput Assist Tomogr 1997;21:773–9.
6. Tan JE, Orel SG, Schnall MD, et al. Role of magnetic resonance imaging and magnetic resonance imaging-guided surgery in the evaluation of patients with early-stage breast cancer for breast conservation treatment. Am J Clin Oncol 1999;22:414–8.
7. Berg WA, Gutierrez L, NessAiver MS, et al. Diagnostic accuracy of mammography, clinical examination, US, and MR imaging in preoperative assessment of breast cancer 1. Radiology 2004; 233:830–49.
8. Boetes C, Mus R, Holland R, et al. Breast tumors: comparative accuracy of MR imaging relative to mammography and US for demonstrating extent. Radiology 1995;197:743–7.
9. American College of Radiology. ACR practice guideline for the performance of contrast-enhanced magnetic resonance imaging (MRI) of the breast. Reston (VA): American College of Radiology; 2008.
10. Mauri D, Pavlidis N, Ioannidis JP. Neoadjuvant versus adjuvant systemic treatment in breast cancer: a meta-analysis. J Natl Cancer Inst 2005;97: 188–94.
11. Abrial SC, Penault-Llorca F, Delva R, et al. High prognostic significance of residual disease after neoadjuvant chemotherapy: a retrospective study in 710 patients with operable breast cancer. Breast Cancer Res Treat 2005;94:255–63.
12. Houssami N, Ciatto S, Macaskill P, et al. Accuracy and surgical impact of magnetic resonance imaging in breast cancer staging: systematic review and meta-analysis in detection of multifocal and multicentric cancer. J Clin Oncol 2008;26:3248–58.
13. Iacconi C, Galman L, Zheng J, et al. Multicentric cancer detected at breast MR imaging and not at mammography: important or not? Radiology 2015; 279:378–84.
14. Plana MN, Carreira C, Muriel A, et al. Magnetic resonance imaging in the preoperative assessment of patients with primary breast cancer: systematic review of diagnostic accuracy and meta-analysis. Eur Radiol 2012;22:26–38.
15. Brennan ME, Houssami N, Lord S, et al. Magnetic resonance imaging screening of the contralateral breast in women with newly diagnosed breast cancer: systematic review and meta-analysis of incremental cancer detection and impact on surgical management. J Clin Oncol 2009;27:5640–9.
16. Bufi E, Belli P, Di Matteo M, et al. Hypervascularity predicts complete pathologic response to chemotherapy and late outcomes in breast cancer. Clin Breast Cancer 2016;16:e193–201.
17. Harowicz MR, Saha A, Grimm LJ, et al. Can algorithmically assessed MRI features predict which patients with a preoperative diagnosis of ductal carcinoma in situ are upstaged to invasive breast cancer? J Magn Reson Imaging 2017;46(5):1332–40.
18. De Los Santos JF, Cantor A, Amos KD, et al. Magnetic resonance imaging as a predictor of pathologic response in patients treated with neoadjuvant systemic treatment for operable breast cancer. Cancer 2013;119:1776–83.
19. Golden DI, Lipson JA, Telli ML, et al. Dynamic contrast-enhanced MRI-based biomarkers of therapeutic response in triple-negative breast cancer. J Am Med Inform Assoc 2013;20:1059–66.
20. Uematsu T, Kasami M, Yuen S. Triple-negative breast cancer: correlation between MR imaging and pathologic findings 1. Radiology 2009;250: 638–47.

21. Loo CE, Straver ME, Rodenhuis S, et al. Magnetic resonance imaging response monitoring of breast cancer during neoadjuvant chemotherapy: relevance of breast cancer subtype. J Clin Oncol 2011;29:660–6.

22. Hayashi Y, Takei H, Nozu S, et al. Analysis of complete response by MRI following neoadjuvant chemotherapy predicts pathological tumor responses differently for molecular subtypes of breast cancer. Corrigendum in/ol/5/4/1433. Oncol Lett 2013;5:83–9.

23. DeMartini W, Lehman C, Partridge S. Breast MRI for cancer detection and characterization: a review of evidence-based clinical applications. Acad Radiol 2008;15:408–16.

24. Martincich L, Montemurro F, De Rosa G, et al. Monitoring response to primary chemotherapy in breast cancer using dynamic contrast-enhanced magnetic resonance imaging. Breast Cancer Res Treat 2004; 83:67–76.

25. Pickles MD, Lowry M, Manton DJ, et al. Role of dynamic contrast enhanced MRI in monitoring early response of locally advanced breast cancer to neoadjuvant chemotherapy. Breast Cancer Res Treat 2005;91:1–10.

26. Padhani AR, Hayes C, Assersohn L, et al. Prediction of clinicopathologic response of breast cancer to primary chemotherapy at contrast-enhanced MR imaging: initial clinical results 1. Radiology 2006;239: 361–74.

27. Cheung Y-C, Chen S-C, Su M-Y, et al. Monitoring the size and response of locally advanced breast cancers to neoadjuvant chemotherapy (weekly paclitaxel and epirubicin) with serial enhanced MRI. Breast Cancer Res Treat 2003;78:51–8.

28. Manton D, Chaturvedi A, Hubbard A, et al. Neoadjuvant chemotherapy in breast cancer: early response prediction with quantitative MR imaging and spectroscopy. Br J Cancer 2006;94:427–35.

29. Wasser K, Klein S, Fink C, et al. Evaluation of neoadjuvant chemotherapeutic response of breast cancer using dynamic MRI with high temporal resolution. Eur Radiol 2003;13:80–7.

30. Murata Y, Ogawa Y, Yoshida S, et al. Utility of initial MRI for predicting extent of residual disease after neoadjuvant chemotherapy: analysis of 70 breast cancer patients. Oncol Rep 2004;12:1257–62.

31. Esserman L, Kaplan E, Partridge S, et al. MRI phenotype is associated with response to doxorubicin and cyclophosphamide neoadjuvant chemotherapy in stage III breast cancer. Ann Surg Oncol 2001;8:549–59.

32. Yeh E, Slanetz P, Kopans DB, et al. Prospective comparison of mammography, sonography, and MRI in patients undergoing neoadjuvant chemotherapy for palpable breast cancer. AJR Am J Roentgenol 2005;184:868–77.

33. Shin H, Kim H, Ahn J, et al. Comparison of mammography, sonography, MRI and clinical examination in patients with locally advanced or inflammatory breast cancer who underwent neoadjuvant chemotherapy. Br J Radiol 2011;84(1003):612–20.

34. Rigter LS, Loo CE, Linn SC, et al. Neoadjuvant chemotherapy adaptation and serial MRI response monitoring in ER-positive HER2-negative breast cancer. Br J Cancer 2013;109:2965–72.

35. Loo CE, Teertstra HJ, Rodenhuis S, et al. Dynamic contrast-enhanced MRI for prediction of breast cancer response to neoadjuvant chemotherapy: initial results. AJR Am J Roentgenol 2008;191:1331–8.

36. Li W, Arasu V, Newitt DC, et al. Effect of MR imaging contrast thresholds on prediction of neoadjuvant chemotherapy response in breast cancer subtypes: a subgroup analysis of the ACRIN 6657/I-SPY 1 TRIAL. Tomography 2016;2:378.

37. Partridge SC, Gibbs JE, Lu Y, et al. MRI measurements of breast tumor volume predict response to neoadjuvant chemotherapy and recurrence-free survival. AJR Am J Roentgenol 2005;184:1774–81.

38. Choi JS, Ko ES, Ko EY, et al. Background parenchymal enhancement on preoperative magnetic resonance imaging: association with recurrence-free survival in breast cancer patients treated with neoadjuvant chemotherapy. Medicine (Baltimore) 2016;95(9):e3000.

39. Pujara AC, Raad RA, Ponzo F, et al. Standardized uptake values from PET/MRI in metastatic breast cancer: an organ-based comparison with PET/CT. Breast J 2016;22(3):264–73.

40. Costelloe CM, Rohren EM, Madewell JE, et al. Imaging bone metastases in breast cancer: techniques and recommendations for diagnosis. Lancet Oncol 2009;10:606–14.

41. O'Sullivan GJ, Carty FL, Cronin CG. Imaging of bone metastasis: an update. World J Radiol 2015;7:202.

42. Qayyum A, MacVicar AD, Padhani AR, et al. Symptomatic brachial plexopathy following treatment for breast cancer: utility of MR imaging with surface-coil techniques 1. Radiology 2000;214:837–42.

43. Scott BJ, Kesari S. Leptomeningeal metastases in breast cancer. Am J Cancer Res 2013;3:117–26.

44. De Bresser J, De Vos B, Van der Ent F, et al. Breast MRI in clinically and mammographically occult breast cancer presenting with an axillary metastasis: a systematic review. Eur J Surg Oncol 2010;36: 114–9.

How Does MR Imaging Help Care for My Breast Cancer Patient? Perspective of a Radiation Oncologist

Kaitlin M. Christopherson, MD[a], Benjamin D. Smith, MD[b],*

KEYWORDS

- Partial breast radiotherapy • MR imaging • Breast cancer

KEY POINTS

- For patients with preinvasive breast cancer or early-stage breast cancer, MR imaging may help identify patients who are eligible for accelerated partial breast irradiation.
- In early-stage patients, MR imaging may provide benefit in accuracy and consistency of target volume delineation for radiation treatment planning, particularly in the preoperative setting.
- In select patients, MR imaging may identify extramammary disease that alters the overall treatment recommendation, target volumes, and/or doses of radiation therapy.
- MR imaging is capable of showing late sequela of radiation in patients with breast cancer and may have a role in examining late breast fibrosis in future studies.

INTRODUCTION

Radiation therapy (RT) can be used in almost every stage of breast cancer. In preinvasive and early-stage invasive breast cancer, radiation is used in the adjuvant setting after breast-conserving surgery. For advanced-stage patients, radiation may be indicated to treat regional nodal basins and the chest wall following mastectomy and axillary surgery. Even in stage IV disease, there is recently increased interest in aggressive local therapy, particularly in patients with limited metastases (oligometastatic cancer).

The general guiding principles of radiation include targeting malignancies while sparing normal adjacent tissue from high-dose radiation. To achieve the maximal balance between efficacy and morbidity, it is critically important to accurately define the radiation target. Current practice relies heavily on the utility of computed tomography (CT)-based radiation treatment planning. In the United States, CT-based simulation scans, or treatment planning scans, are the most commonly used planning method for radiation oncologists. On these images, the radiation oncologist defines the target, also referred to as the clinical treatment volume, and defines nearby organs at risk to avoid.

Given the range of possible radiation treatments in breast cancer, MR imaging has several possible applications for the radiation oncologist. Herein, the authors focus on the usefulness of MR imaging for the radiation oncologist in the setting of both early-stage disease and late-stage

Disclosure Statement: The authors have nothing to disclose.
[a] Department of Radiation Oncology, The University of Texas MD Anderson Cancer Center, Boone Pickens Academic Tower (FCT6.5075), 1515 Holcombe Boulevard, Houston, TX 77030, USA; [b] Department of Radiation Oncology, The University of Texas MD Anderson Cancer Center, Unit 1202, 1515 Holcombe Boulevard, Houston, TX 77030, USA
* Corresponding author.
E-mail address: Bsmith3@mdanderson.org

Magn Reson Imaging Clin N Am 26 (2018) 295–302
https://doi.org/10.1016/j.mric.2017.12.007
1064-9689/18/© 2017 Elsevier Inc. All rights reserved.

disease. For early-stage patients, MR imaging can aid in target delineation and radiation technique selection. For more advanced-stage patients, this article examines how MR imaging may help identify the extent of disease in addition to aid in target volume definition. Last, the authors comment on MR imaging in monitoring of late effects of radiation.

EARLY-STAGE PATIENTS

In early-stage and preinvasive cancers, radiation is used in conjunction with lumpectomy to minimize the risk of subsequent in-breast tumor recurrence and thus maximize the likelihood of breast conservation long-term survival. The most common radiation approach in early-stage disease is whole breast irradiation (WBI), in which tangential radiation beams are directed from the medial and lateral aspects of the affected breast for a series of daily treatments ranging from approximately 3 to 6 weeks (Fig. 1). A tumor bed boost, defined as additional radiation directed to the tissues immediately adjacent to the tumor bed, is frequently delivered following WBI to further lower local recurrence risks. Multiple randomized trials have demonstrated that lumpectomy followed by WBI confers survival equivalent to mastectomy, and as such, WBI is a commonly accepted standard of care.[1–5] Accelerated partial breast irradiation (APBI) is a newer approach to delivery of radiation for breast cancer, in which only tissues immediately adjacent to the tumor bed are targeted and treated with radiation (Fig. 2). Currently, use of APBI is largely limited to women age ≥50 years with estrogen receptor–positive, node-negative tumors measuring 2 cm or less in size.[6]

Within the context of WBI and APBI, MR imaging has several important potential applications. First, by detecting the presence or absence of radiographically occult disease in the breast that is remote from the tumor bed, MR imaging can assist in determining which patients may be safely treated with APBI and which patients would be better served by WBI (or even mastectomy). Second, because of better soft tissue resolution than typically achieved with radiation planning CT scans, MR imaging may assist with delineation of the tumor bed to enhance treatment planning of APBI or the tumor bed boost. Third, recent investigations have focused on developing novel preoperative APBI treatment strategies, and in this setting, MR imaging can be invaluable in identifying the in vivo tumor and facilitating accurate targeting with radiation before surgery. Each of these important scenarios is discussed in detail in later discussion.

Patient Selection for Accelerated Partial Breast Irradiation

For early-stage patients who may be candidates for APBI, breast MR imaging may be of value to the radiation oncologist by identifying the presence of malignant foci remote from the tumor bed, which, if present, would disqualify the patient from being eligible for APBI.[7–10] For example, Tendulkar and colleagues[8] reviewed 260 patients with early breast cancer treated at the Cleveland Clinic and correlated findings on mammography, MR imaging, and surgical pathology. The objective was to determine if MR imaging was more sensitive than mammography in patient selection for APBI. They focused on patients who would have been eligible for National Surgical Adjuvant Breast and Bowel Project B-39 (a prospective trial evaluating APBI) based on clinical-pathologic grounds. MR imaging detected synchronous, mammographically occult, primaries in 5.8% of patients, most commonly in the ipsilateral breast. They noted that invasive lobular carcinoma (ILC), in contrast to invasive ductal carcinoma, was significantly associated with additional ipsilateral disease (18% of these patients).

A similar study from the University of Chicago prospectively evaluated the benefit of MR imaging for more than 500 patients being screened for APBI and concluded that preoperative breast MR imaging rendered 12.9% of patient ineligible for APBI. Risk factors for ineligibility included tumor size ≥2 cm, age less than 50, ILC, and Her-2/neu amplification. A combination of these factors was used to generate a risk score that predicted the likelihood that MR imaging would render a patient ineligible for APBI.[9]

In total, these and other studies indicate that preoperative MR imaging could alter recommendations for partial breast irradiation in up to 13% of patients. Most commonly, MR images reveal more extensive ipsilateral disease or multifocality, but can also detect contralateral breast lesions as well.[10–14] Known multifocal or multicentric disease would be a contraindication for APBI. It is important to take into account certain clinical and pathologic factors, such as young age, tumor size, and invasive lobular histology, which may lead to a higher yield of additional findings on breast MR imaging. For a young patient with ILC, or a patient with a 2-cm or greater tumor, who is motivated for APBI, it may be reasonable to consider breast MR imaging to rule out possible multifocal or multicentric ipsilateral disease.[14,15]

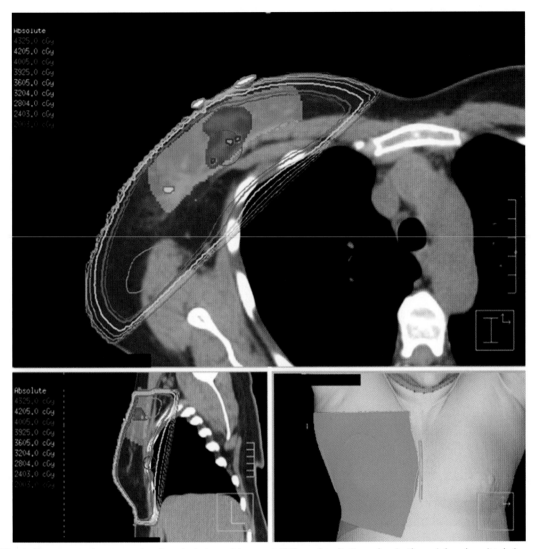

Fig. 1. Representative example of a whole breast tangent CT-based radiation plan in the axial and sagittal views. The red volume is the volume defined as tumor bed. Skin rendering is also shown. (*Courtesy of* Elizabeth Bloom, MD, Houston, TX.)

Postoperative Delineation for Accelerated Partial Breast Irradiation or External Beam Boost

For patients with an indication for postoperative radiation, treatment planning usually begins with a CT simulation scan 3 to 6 weeks after surgery. At the time of simulation, the radiation oncologist contours the tumor bed based on soft tissue change seen on CT and radiopaque clips left by the surgeon to mark the tumor bed. This contour is critically important, because it will be used to delineate the treatment volume for either APBI or, in the setting of WBI, the external beam tumor bed boost. Accurate delineation of the tumor bed is critical to achieve optimal radiotherapy outcomes. Failure to delineate the entirety of the tumor bed could lead to higher risk of local failure, because volumes at risk for recurrence that are not delineated could harbor residual disease that would not be adequately treated. Conversely, inclusion of non–tumor bed tissue within the tumor bed contour results in a larger volume of radiated tissue, which may yield increased late risks of soft tissue fibrosis and/or suboptimal cosmetic outcome. In consideration of the importance of accurate tumor bed delineation, various groups have investigated the utility of MR image fusion with CT-based radiation treatment planning to improve accuracy of tumor bed delineation. MR imaging obtained in the treatment position may be fused in the radiation planning software to aid in

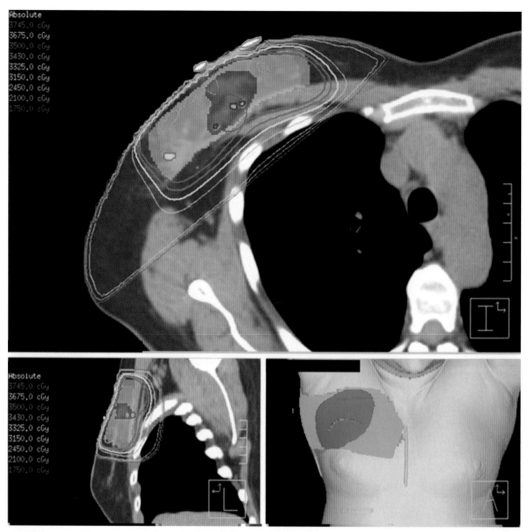

Fig. 2. Representative example of partial breast CT-based radiation plan. The red volume represents the tumor bed contour, and the aqua volume represents a volumetric expansion of 2.0 cm around the tumor bed to create a clinical treatment volume. Skin rendering is also shown. (*Courtesy of* Elizabeth Bloom, MD, Houston, TX.)

contouring of the tumor bed. MR image fusions for radiation therapy target volume delineation have proven useful in other disease sites, such as the central nervous system, head and neck, sarcoma, genitourinary, and gynecologic cancers, so it is reasonable to posit that a similar approach could be useful for breast cancer.

A study from Jolicoeur and colleagues[16] evaluated the value of postoperative MR image fusion to CT-based planning for brachytherapy planning in the supine treatment position. They evaluated the accuracy of contours between practitioners. Consistency in target volume definition is typically measured as interobserver variability, with more accuracy correlating to low variability. The use of MR fusion led to a reduction in the volume of tumor bed contoured by 30% to 40% with little

interobserver variability.[16] Although this study is promising and potentially clinically meaningful, other similar studies have reported discordant findings regarding the usefulness of MR image fusion with CT-based treatment planning scans.[16–20] In light of the conflicting evidence, at this time the authors' group does not routinely obtain MR imaging to assist in tumor bed delineation, although it may be considered in rare cases whereby tumor bed delineation is critically important and CT-based imaging is difficult to interpret.

Defining the Preoperative Accelerated Partial Breast Irradiation Target

As previously mentioned, RT is most commonly delivered postoperatively after breast surgery.

There are inherent difficulties associated with this method because of seroma and/or hematoma formation that may enlarge the radiated volume, and variability of clip placement around the tumor bed cavity. In other disease sites, such as soft tissue sarcomas, esophageal, and rectal cancers, radiotherapy is used preoperatively.[21–23] Preoperative radiation has certain advantages, principally the potential to facilitate smaller treatment volumes and lower doses of radiation. Disadvantages include risks of impaired wound healing postoperatively. Recent emerging literature has sought to define the role of preoperative radiotherapy for patients with breast cancer in an effort to mitigate some of the inherent difficulties related to postoperative treatment planning. These studies focus on contouring accuracy to ensure tumor coverage, without excess normal tissue exposure to RT, with ultimate goals of reducing late toxicities.

A study by den Hartogh and colleagues[24] examined preoperative tumor delineation on both CT and MR imaging for patients undergoing breast-conserving surgery. The study sought to quantify the consistency of preoperative tumor delineation among 4 observers. When delineating gross tumor, there was high interobserver agreement for both CT and MR images. Contours obtained from MR images resulted in larger contours (compared with CT based), because MR images were able to show details of more irregularly shaped and spiculated tumors. Despite this fact, when comparing both CT and MR preoperative tumor volumes with postoperative tumor bed volumes in other studies, both sets of preoperative tumor volumes were considerably smaller. These findings suggest that preoperative MR-guided APBI may allow for more accurate and precise treatment volumes.

Preoperative partial breast radiation is not used off-protocol at present, but there is ongoing investigation in this arena. Modern protocols for preoperative partial breast radiotherapy commonly use MR images to aid in target delineation and thus treatment planning. As radiation oncologists, the authors look forward to emerging data regarding the efficacy and safety of this treatment approach.

ADVANCED-STAGE PATIENTS

In more advanced breast cancer cases, radiation may be necessary after mastectomy, axillary surgery, and chemotherapy to decrease the risk for local-regional recurrence and improve disease-specific survival.[25–27] For patients with node-positive and locally advanced cancers, it is important to accurately determine the extent of disease at initial presentation as well as the final pathologic stage, when determining radiation treatment volumes and doses. Of the routine breast imaging modalities, MR imaging is the only modality that routinely encompasses extramammary sites in the examination. For radiation oncologists, extramammary findings that could alter treatment recommendations include those representing locally advanced disease, such as internal mammary (IM) or mediastinal adenopathy, skin involvement, and sternal involvement. For widely metastatic disease, radiation may play no role. MR findings may upstage a patient, emphasizing the need for accurate and detailed preoperative imaging, whereby MR imaging may provide information that would not be available from mammography or ultrasound in primary breast cancer staging.

Identification of Locally Advanced Disease: Extensive Lymphatic Spread/Sternal Involvement

Bones of the chest wall, lungs, liver, and additional nodal stations can be seen on some breast MR images depending on the institution's set scan range. Up to one-third of breast MR images show extramammary findings.[28] Most extramammary findings are benign, but 10% to 20% are malignant, with a higher likelihood of malignancy in patients undergoing MR imaging for staging of a known invasive cancer.[28–30] Knowing that the most common sites of metastases in breast cancer are lymph nodes and bone, careful attention to draining nodal basins, ribs, sternum, and spine on breast MR imaging may reveal additional disease. Additional findings in these locations may contribute to staging and prognosis. Enlarged IM nodes can readily be seen on breast MR imaging as enhancing nodal masses (Fig. 3). IM involvement obviously alters the stage of the breast cancer, and invariably, patients with IM involvement will require trimodality treatment. Because the IM nodes are rarely dissected at surgery, this nodal

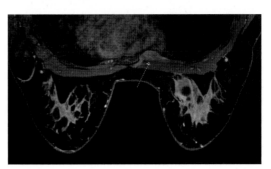

Fig. 3. MR imaging showing pathologic left-sided IM (*arrow*) adenopathy.

chain must be treated with relatively high doses of radiation to yield long-term local-regional control. Breast MR imaging can be useful to the radiation oncologist to follow response to chemotherapy of a positive IM node and may influence volume of IM nodal basin covered with radiation and the final radiation dose delivered. An isolated sternal lesion may be noted on staging MR imaging (**Fig. 4**), and subsequently targeted with postoperative radiation in select patients with oligometastatic disease.

Identification of Locally Advanced Disease: Skin Thickening/Inflammatory Breast Cancer

In primary tumor staging, skin involvement leads to a stage T4 diagnosis and requires more local-regional treatment. Skin involvement is typically regarded as a physical examination finding, but MR images can also identify skin involvement on initial staging of a patient with breast cancer and can serve to clarify equivocal findings on examination.[29] Inflammatory breast cancer (IBC) is the most aggressive form of breast cancer, characterized by physical examination findings of skin redness and edema. Although clinical features are necessary to confirm IBC diagnosis, MR imaging can support a clinician's examination findings. The National Comprehensive Cancer Network guidelines recommend optional MR imaging in the staging of patients with IBC. MR imaging can elucidate inflammatory changes in the breasts by showing skin changes in conjunction with edema

and detects skin edema more often than mammography.[31] MR imaging can be particularly helpful in the setting of patients with clinical features of IBC in the absence of a readily defined breast mass on conventional mammography and ultrasound. Patients with inflammatory presentation are also more likely to have regional nodal or distant spread, so MR imaging can be useful to outline the full extent of disease before initiation of any therapy. In the evaluation of IBC, an MR imaging examination can clearly show an asymmetrically large breast, with thickened skin edema and sometimes diffuse involvement of the affected breast (**Fig. 5**).

RADIATION SIDE EFFECTS

Radiation can lead to long-term tissue changes and the potential for side effects. For patients with breast cancer, late effects can include breast and lung fibrosis, which result in clinically symptomatic side effects in the minority of patients.

As mentioned previously, standard whole breast or post–mastectomy radiation involves using tangential fields to treat the whole breast or chest wall and invariably requires radiation beams to pass through the lung immediately posterior to the chest wall (typically on the order of 2 cm depth of lung). Treating this small strip of lung rarely leads to symptomatic clinical complaints for patients, but more commonly does result in radiographic lung changes. In subsequent breast MR images after breast cancer treatment radiation, fibrosis in this area can be visualized as a subpleural linear band of enhancement.[29]

There is also interest in quantifying radiation-induced breast fibrosis, especially as it related to quality of life and cosmetic outcomes. A study from Hammer and colleagues[32] found the volume

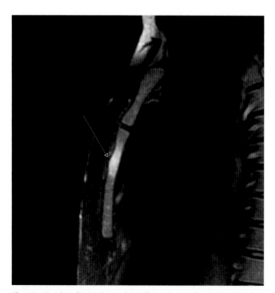

Fig. 4. Sagittal MR imaging showing enhancing lesion in the sternum (*arrow*). This finding was noted for a patient undergoing initial evaluation for what was thought to be stage II breast cancer.

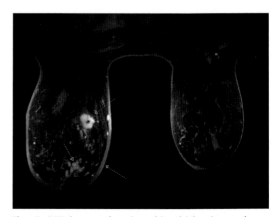

Fig. 5. MR image showing skin thickening, edema, and multiple foci of enhancement (*arrows*) in a patient diagnosed with right-sided IBC.

of breast tissue receiving ≥ 55 Gy correlated with rates of grade 2 fibrosis. If MR imaging can be optimized to more accurately identify the tumor bed and minimize boost volumes compared with CT, this could prove useful in potentially reducing late fibrosis. There have been few published studies on the value of MR imaging in assessing the degree of post-RT fibrosis. MR elastography is a tool used to measure stiffness in soft tissues and may prove useful in the future in quantifying post-RT breast fibrosis.[33]

SUMMARY

MR imaging can assist the radiation oncologist in patients with both early and advanced disease breast cancer. Radiation oncologists thus need to evaluate MR breast images, when obtained, to ensure that these imaging findings are taken into consideration when developing a radiation therapy management plan. Future research may establish a definitive role for MR imaging in facilitating preoperative partial breast radiation therapy and in quantitatively measuring the extent of postradiation soft tissue toxicity.

REFERENCES

1. Blichert-Toft M, Nielsen M, Düring M, et al. Long-term results of breast conserving surgery vs. mastectomy for early stage invasive breast cancer: 20-year follow-up of the Danish randomized DBCG-82TM protocol. Acta Oncol 2008;47(4):672–81.
2. Simone NL, Dan T, Shih J, et al. Twenty-five year results of the National Cancer Institute randomized breast conservation trial. Breast Cancer Res Treat 2012;132(1):197–203.
3. Litière S, Werutsky G, Fentiman IS, et al. Breast conserving therapy versus mastectomy for stage I-II breast cancer: 20 year follow-up of the EORTC 10801 phase 3 randomised trial. Lancet Oncol 2012;13(4):412–9.
4. Fisher B, Anderson S, Bryant J, et al. Twenty-year follow-up of a randomized trial comparing total mastectomy, lumpectomy, and lumpectomy plus irradiation for the treatment of invasive breast cancer. N Engl J Med 2002;347(16):1233–41.
5. Early Breast Cancer Trialists' Collaborative Group (EBCTCG), Darby S, McGale P, Correa C, et al. Effect of radiotherapy after breast-conserving surgery on 10-year recurrence and 15-year breast cancer death: meta-analysis of individual patient data for 10,801 women in 17 randomised trials. Lancet 2011;378(9804):1707–16.
6. Correa C, Harris EE, Leonardi MC, et al. Accelerated partial breast irradiation: executive summary for the update of an ASTRO evidence-based consensus statement. Pract Radiat Oncol 2017;7(2):73–9.
7. Al-Hallaq HA, Mell LK, Bradley JA, et al. Magnetic resonance imaging identifies multifocal and multi-centric disease in breast cancer patients who are eligible for partial breast irradiation. Cancer 2008;113(9):2408–14.
8. Tendulkar RD, Chellman-Jeffers M, Rybicki LA, et al. Preoperative breast magnetic resonance imaging in early breast cancer: implications for partial breast irradiation. Cancer 2009;115(8):1621–30.
9. Dorn PL, Al-Hallaq HA, Haq F, et al. A prospective study of the utility of magnetic resonance imaging in determining candidacy for partial breast irradiation. Int J Radiat Oncol Biol Phys 2013;85(3):615–22.
10. Tallet A, Rua S, Jalaguier A, et al. Impact of preoperative magnetic resonance imaging in breast cancer patients candidates for an intraoperative partial breast irradiation. Transl Cancer Res 2015;4(2):148–54.
11. Schnall MD, Blume J, Bluemke DA, et al. MRI detection of distinct incidental cancer in women with primary breast cancer studied in IBMC 6883. J Surg Oncol 2005;92(1):32–8.
12. Gutierrez RL, DeMartini WB, Silbergeld JJ, et al. High cancer yield and positive predictive value: outcomes at a center routinely using preoperative breast MRI for staging. AJR Am J Roentgenol 2011;196(1):W93–9.
13. Kowalchik KV, Vallow LA, McDonough M, et al. The role of preoperative bilateral breast magnetic resonance imaging in patient selection for partial breast irradiation in ductal carcinoma in situ. Int J Surg Oncol 2012;2012:206342.
14. Kowalchik KV, Vallow LA, McDonough M, et al. Classification system for identifying women at risk for altered partial breast irradiation recommendations after breast magnetic resonance imaging. Int J Radiat Oncol Biol Phys 2013;87(1):127–33.
15. Houssami N, Turner R, Morrow M. Preoperative magnetic resonance imaging in breast cancer: meta-analysis of surgical outcomes. Ann Surg 2013;257(2):249–55.
16. Jolicoeur M, Racine ML, Trop I, et al. Localization of the surgical bed using supine magnetic resonance and computed tomography scan fusion for planification of breast interstitial brachytherapy. Radiother Oncol 2011;100(3):480–4.
17. Kirby AM, Yarnold JR, Evans PM, et al. Tumor bed delineation for partial breast and breast boost radiotherapy planned in the prone position: what does MRI add to X-ray CT localization of titanium clips placed in the excision cavity wall? Int J Radiat Oncol Biol Phys 2009;74(4):1276–82.
18. Giezen M, Kouwenhoven E, Scholten AN, et al. MRI-versus CT-based volume delineation of lumpectomy

cavity in supine position in breast-conserving therapy: an exploratory study. Int J Radiat Oncol Biol Phys 2012;82(4):1332–40.

19. Huang W, Currey A, Chen X, et al. A comparison of lumpectomy cavity delineations between use of magnetic resonance imaging and computed tomography acquired with patient in prone position for radiation therapy planning of breast cancer. Int J Radiat Oncol Biol Phys 2016;94(4):832–40.

20. Mast M, Coerkamp E, Heijenbrok M, et al. Target volume delineation in breast conserving radiotherapy: are co-registered CT and MR images of added value? Radiat Oncol 2014;9:65.

21. Davis AM, O'Sullivan B, Turcotte R, et al. Late radiation morbidity following randomization to preoperative versus postoperative radiotherapy in extremity soft tissue sarcoma. Radiother Oncol 2005;75(1): 48–53.

22. Sauer R, Liersch T, Merkel S, et al. Preoperative versus postoperative chemoradiotherapy for locally advanced rectal cancer: results of the German CAO/ARO/AIO-94 randomized phase III trial after a median follow-up of 11 years. J Clin Oncol 2012; 30(16):1926–33.

23. Shapiro J, van Lanschot JJB, Hulshof MCCM, et al. Neoadjuvant chemoradiotherapy plus surgery versus surgery alone for oesophageal or junctional cancer (CROSS): long-term results of a randomised controlled trial. Lancet Oncol 2015;16(9):1090–8.

24. den Hartogh MD, Philippens ME, van Dam IE, et al. MRI and CT imaging for preoperative target volume delineation in breast-conserving therapy. Radiat Oncol 2014;9:63.

25. Clarke M, Collins R, Darby S, et al. Effects of radiotherapy and of differences in the extent of surgery for early breast cancer on local recurrence and 15-year survival: an overview of the randomised trials. Lancet 2005;366(9503):2087–106.

26. Danish Breast Cancer Cooperative Group, Nielsen HM, Overgaard M, Grau C, et al. Study of failure pattern among high-risk breast cancer patients with or without postmastectomy radiotherapy in addition to adjuvant systemic therapy: long-term results from the Danish Breast Cancer Cooperative Group DBCG 82 b and c randomized studies. J Clin Oncol 2006;24(15):2268–75.

27. Ragaz J, Olivotto IA, Spinelli JJ, et al. Locoregional radiation therapy in patients with high-risk breast cancer receiving adjuvant chemotherapy: 20-year results of the British Columbia randomized trial. J Natl Cancer Inst 2005;97(2):116–26.

28. Iodice D, Di Donato O, Liccardo I, et al. Prevalence of extramammary findings on breast MRI: a large retrospective single-centre study. Radiol Med 2013;118(7):1109–18.

29. Gao Y, Ibidapo O, Toth HK, et al. Delineating extramammary findings at breast MR imaging. Radiographics 2017;37(1):10–31.

30. Rinaldi P, Costantini M, Belli P, et al. Extra-mammary findings in breast MRI. Eur Radiol 2011;21(11): 2268–76.

31. Girardi V, Carbognin G, Camera L, et al. Inflammatory breast carcinoma and locally advanced breast carcinoma: characterisation with MR imaging. Radiol Med 2011;116(1):71–83.

32. Hammer C, Maduro JH, Bantema-Joppe EJ, et al. Radiation-induced fibrosis in the boost area after three-dimensional conformal radiotherapy with a simultaneous integrated boost technique for early-stage breast cancer: a multivariable prediction model. Radiother Oncol 2017;122(1):45–9.

33. Hawley JR, Kalra P, Mo X, et al. Quantification of breast stiffness using MR elastography at 3 Tesla with a soft sternal driver: a reproducibility study. J Magn Reson Imaging 2017;45(5):1379–84.

American College of Radiology Accreditation, Performance Metrics, Reimbursement, and Economic Considerations in Breast MR Imaging

Matthew F. Covington, MD, Catherine A. Young, MD, JD, Catherine M. Appleton, MD*

KEYWORDS

• Breast MR Imaging • ACR accreditation • Performance metrics • Reimbursement • Economics

KEY POINTS

- Medicare and many private insurers require breast MR imaging to be performed by an accredited facility for an examination to be eligible for reimbursement.
- The Breast Magnetic Resonance Imaging Accreditation Program (BMRAP) offered by the American College of Radiology (ACR) is a comprehensive quality assurance program that provides facilities with peer review and feedback.
- In addition to adherence to technical practice parameters and quality control standards, facilities must have a medical outcomes audit program for accreditation by the ACR BMRAP.
- Although screening breast MR imaging is currently only considered cost-effective for women at high risk of developing breast cancer, cost-competition and abbreviated protocols could increase its cost-effectiveness for women at lower risk levels.

INTRODUCTION

Imaging centers performing breast MR imaging in the United States must be accredited to qualify for reimbursement from Medicare and many private insurers. The only pathway to accreditation at this time is through the American College of Radiology (ACR) Breast Magnetic Resonance Imaging Accreditation Program (BMRAP). The BMRAP is a comprehensive quality assurance program designed to ensure technical quality and promote interpretive quality throughout the industry. To aid breast imagers, the requirements and process for BMRAP accreditation are outlined in this article, followed by a discussion of medical outcomes monitoring as a vital quality assurance tool. Finally, important economic considerations for performance of breast MR imaging are presented.

ACCREDITATION OVERVIEW
Background

Founded in 1923, the ACR is a professional medical organization committed to advancing the

Disclosure Statement: The authors have nothing to disclose.
Mallinckrodt Institute of Radiology, Washington University School of Medicine, 510 South Kingshighway Boulevard, Saint Louis, MO 63110, USA
* Corresponding author.
E-mail address: appletonc@wustl.edu

Magn Reson Imaging Clin N Am 26 (2018) 303–314
https://doi.org/10.1016/j.mric.2017.12.004
1064-9689/18/© 2018 Elsevier Inc. All rights reserved.

"practice, science and professions of radiologic care."[1] With stated core values including leadership, quality, integrity, and innovation, the college is organized around 5 pillars: economics, advocacy, education, quality and safety, and clinical research. In the realm of quality and safety, the ACR has a rich history of accreditation, beginning in 1986 with radiation oncology.[2] A year later, mammography accreditation began and gained broad acceptance among facilities.[3] To ensure access to high-quality mammography, the US Food and Drug Administration subsequently adopted the ACR mammography accreditation program by enacting the Mammography Quality Standards Act of 1992 (MQSA).[4] The ACR has since developed other imaging accreditation programs; at present, there are at least 36,000 ACR-accredited facilities among the various programs.[1]

In 2010, the ACR launched its BMRAP,[5] and it remains the only pathway to accreditation in the United States. The BRMAP sets forth minimum standards for performing high-quality breast MR imaging. It not only specifies technical practice parameters but also required training and qualifications for personnel, equipment, and maintenance and quality-control/assurance measures. There are fees for initial accreditation, accreditation of additional units, repeat testing, reinstatement or corrective action plans, and replacement certificates.[6] Through the accreditation process, the BMRAP provides facilities with peer review and constructive feedback concerning their breast MR imaging programs.[6] As of January 1, 2016, accreditation in all voluntary breast imaging accreditation programs, including MR imaging, is necessary for the designation ACR Breast Imaging Center of Excellence.

Personnel

All technologists, medical physicists, and interpreting radiologists must meet specific requirements to achieve and maintain accreditation through BMRAP. The respective qualifications are detailed in **Tables 1–3**.

Technical Considerations

The BMRAP is unit based. Each individual unit used for diagnostic imaging must pass accreditation for a facility to achieve accreditation. Regular preventative maintenance is required and must be performed by a qualified service engineer. Although there is no requirement for magnet field strength, units must have a dedicated breast coil capable of simultaneous bilateral imaging. Bilateral imaging is superior for several reasons: it allows for comparison of both breasts, including evaluation of background glandular enhancement; identification of

contralateral malignancy in the setting of a known malignancy; and minimizing the possibility of aliasing artifact that might occur in unilateral imaging.[5] Equipment must meet relevant state and federal performance requirements, including those for

- Maximum static magnetic field strength
- Maximum rate of change of magnetic field strength (dB/dt)
- Maximum radiofrequency power deposition (specific absorption rate)
- Maximum auditory noise levels

Facilities must have the ability to execute multimodality breast imaging correlation with mammography, breast ultrasound, and MR imaging–guided breast biopsy. If a facility does not provide biopsy services, it must have an arrangement with another institution, preferably one that is accredited, so that follow-up care can be provided when appropriate.

The ACR publishes practice guidelines and technical standards, which are excellent references for imaging and practice development. Facilities seeking accreditation must comply with the ACR quality control (QC) requirements. Compliance must be documented and performed in accordance with the minimum frequencies included in the most current ACR QC manual provided to the supervising physician. Considerations include acceptance testing, an annual survey by the medical physicist/MR imaging scientist, and technologist QC tests.

Peer Review

The ACR accreditation process requires submission of clinical images for peer review. Facilities are instructed to submit a case of a known biopsy-proved malignancy in an examination demonstrating the facility's best work. Because accreditation is unit specific, a qualifying examination must be submitted for each scanner performing breast MR imaging at any given facility. Submitted images and test image data forms should be approved by the lead interpreting physician.

Once received by the ACR, images are independently reviewed and scored by a qualified physicist and 2 clinical imaging reviewers. Clinical imaging reviewers must be board certified radiologists with at least 5 years of breast MR imaging experience as well as ongoing clinical engagement with the modality; they are also subject to specific continuing medical education requirements. Reviewers score cases on the following categories: pulse sequence and image contrast, positioning and anatomic coverage, artifacts, spatial and temporal resolution, and examination identification. Pass or fail, specific feedback from the evaluation

Table 1		
Radiologist qualifications		
Qualifications	**Radiologist**	**Other Physician**

Initial	Board certified
	• Certification in radiology or diagnostic radiology by the
	  ○ ABR or
	  ○ AOBR or
	  ○ Royal College of Physicians and Surgeons of Canada or
	  ○ Le Collège des médecins du Québec or
	  ○ Radiologist graduating from residency after June 30, 2014, must be board eligible as defined by the ABR
	   AND
	• If board certified before 2008, must also meet 1 of the following:
	  ○ Oversight, interpretation, and reporting of 150 breast MR imaging examinations in the last 36 mo or
	  ○ Interpretation and reporting 100 breast MR imaging examinations in the last 36 mo in a supervised situation
	   AND
	  ○ 15 h of category 1 CME in MR imaging (including clinical applications of MR imaging in breast imaging, MR imaging artifacts, safety, and instrumentation)
	   OR
	Not board certified
	• Completion of an ACGME or AOA approved diagnostic radiology residency program and
	• Interpretation and reporting of 100 breast MR imaging examinations in the last 36 mo in a supervised situation and
	• 15 h of category 1 CME in MR imaging (including clinical applications of MR imaging in breast imaging, MR imaging artifacts, safety, and instrumentation)
		• Completion of an ACGME-approved residency program in the specialty practice and
		• Interpretation and reporting of 300 breast MR imaging examinations in the last 36 mo in a supervised situation and
		• 200 h of category 1 CME in MR imaging (including clinical applications of MR imaging in breast imaging, MR imaging artifacts, safety, and instrumentation)

Continuing experience	On renewal, physicians reading breast MR imaging examinations must meet the following: Currently meet the MOC requirements for ABR (see ABR MOC) or the OCC for AOBR (see AOBR OCC) OR On renewal, *75* breast MR imaging examinations in the prior 36 mo	
Continuing education	On renewal, must meet 1 of the following: 1. Currently meet the MOC requirements for ABR (see ABR MOC) or the OCC for AOBR (see AOBR OCC) OR 2. Complete 150 h (that includes 75 h of category 1 CME) in the prior 36 mo pertinent to the physician's practice patterns (see ACR guideline) OR 3. Completes 15 h CME (half-hours of category 1 CME) in the prior 36 mo specific to the imaging modality or organ system	

Abbreviations: ABR, American Board of Radiology; ACGME, Accreditation Council for Graduate Medical Education; AOA, American Osteopathic Association; AOBR, American Osteopathic Board of Radiology; CME, continuing medical education; MOC, maintenance of certification; OCC, Osteopathic Continuous Certification.

From American College of Radiology. The Breast Magnetic Resonance Imaging (MRI) Accreditation Program Requirements. Available at: http://www.acraccreditation.org/~/media/ACRAccreditation/Documents/Breast-MRI/Requirements.pdf?la=en; with permission.

Table 2
Medical physicist qualifications

Qualifications	Medical Physicist	MR Scientist

Initial	Board certified
	• Certified in diagnostic radiological physics, diagnostic medical physics, or radiological physics by the American Board of Radiology; in diagnostic imaging physics or MR imaging physics by the American Board of Medical Physics, or in diagnostic radiology physics or MR imaging physics by the Canadian College of Physicists in Medicine
	OR
	Not board certified in required subspecialty
	• Graduate degree in medical physics, radiologic physics, physics, or other relevant physical science or engineering discipline from an accredited institution and
	• Formal coursework in the biological sciences with at least
	  ◦ 1 course in biology or radiation biology and
	  ◦ 1 course in anatomy, physiology, or similar topics related to the practice of medical physics
	• 3 y of documented experience in a clinical MR imaging environment
	OR
	Grandfathered
	Conducted surveys of at least 3 MR imaging units between January 1, 2007, and January 1, 2010
		• Graduate degree in a physical science involving nuclear MR or MR imaging
		• 3 y of documented experience in a clinical MR imaging environment

Continuing education	On renewal, *2* MR imaging unit surveys in prior 24 mo	
Continuing education	On renewal, 15 continuing education unit/continuing medical education (1/2 category 1) in prior 36 mo (must include credits pertinent to the accredited modality)	

From American College of Radiology. The Breast Magnetic Resonance Imaging (MRI) Accreditation Program Requirements. Available at: http://www.acraccreditation.org/~/media/ACRAccreditation/Documents/Breast-MRI/Requirements.pdf?la=en; with permission.

is provided to the submitting facility and should be incorporated into its QC, assurance, and improvement efforts.

Specifically, the examination must include

- Localizer/scout sequence
- T2/fluid bright series
- Multiphase T1-weighted precontrast series
- Multiphase T1-weighted early postcontrast series
- Multiphase T1-weighted delayed postcontrast series

Multiphase series should include either fat suppression or subtraction series. The biopsy-proved malignancy must be enhancing and visible on the multiphase postcontrast images. The multiphase precontrast and postcontrast T1 series must have a slice thickness less than or equal to 3 mm, gap of 0 mm, and maximum in-plane pixel dimension for phase and frequency less than or equal to 1 mm.[6] There should be sufficient

signal-to-noise ratio such that the images do not appear grainy. Artifacts should be minimal and should not interfere with the overall diagnostic quality of the examination. Positioning should include the entire breast, including the axillary tail. Unlike mammography, phantom imaging is not currently required for the BMRAP.

Reviewers separately evaluate each examination for accurate identification and labeling, including examination date, patient name (first and last), patient age or date of birth, unique patient identification number, facility name, and laterality. The entire case fails accreditation if the laterality is incorrect or is not included on the images or in the DICOM header. Although the examination report is not part of the clinical image evaluation, in practice, a report is required. This should include the findings with an overall final assessment and recommendation using Breast Imaging Reporting and Data System (BI-RADS) terminology. Mammography, ultrasound, and MR imaging BI-

Table 3
Technologist qualifications

Qualifications	Technologist

Initial	• Registered in MR imaging by the
	  ○ American Registry of Radiologic Technologists or
	  ○ American Registry of Magnetic Resonance Imaging Technologists or
	  ○ Canadian Association of Medical Radiation Technologists
	  OR
	• Registered in radiography by the American Registry of Radiologic Technologists and/or unlimited state license and
	• 6 mo supervised clinical MR imaging scanning experience
	OR
	• Associate degree or bachelor degree in an allied health field and
	• Certification in another clinical imaging field (eg, American Registry for Diagnostic Medical Sonography or Nuclear Medicine Technology Certification Board) and
	• 6 mo supervised clinical MR imaging scanning experience
	AND
	• Licensure in the state in which he/she practices (if required for MR imaging technologists)
	AND
	• Supervised experience in breast MR imaging and
	• Supervised experience in the intravenous administration of MR contrast (if contrast administration is performed by a technologist)

Continuing experience	On renewal, 50 breast MR imaging examinations in the prior 24 mo

Continuing education	• Registered technologists
	  ○ In compliance with the continuing education requirements of their certifying organization for the imaging modality in which they perform services
	  ○ Continuing education includes credits pertinent to the technologist's ACR accredited clinical practice
	• State license technologist
	  ○ 24 h of continuing education every 2 y
	  ○ Continuing education is relevant to imaging and the radiologic sciences, patient care
	  ○ Continuing education includes credits pertinent to the technologist's ACR accredited clinical practice
	• All others
	  ○ 24 h of continuing education every 2 y
	  ○ Continuing education is relevant to imaging and the radiologic sciences, patient care
	  ○ Continuing education includes credits pertinent to the technologist's ACR accredited clinical practice

From American College of Radiology. The Breast Magnetic Resonance Imaging (MRI) Accreditation Program Requirements. Available at: http://www.acraccreditation.org/~/media/ACRAccreditation/Documents/Breast-MRI/Requirements.pdf?la=en; with permission.

RADS lexicons can be found in the *ACR BI-RADS Atlas*,[8] along with definitions and example images. In addition, the *ACR BI-RADS Atlas* provides detailed guidance regarding auditing procedures in its chapter on follow-up and outcome monitoring.

EVALUATING PERFORMANCE
Medical Outcome Audit

Beginning with its original accreditation program for mammography, the ACR has advocated medical outcome monitoring as an essential component of quality assurance. Consequently, the MQSA, which adopted the original ACR mammography accreditation program, mandates that mammography facilities "establish and maintain a mammography medical outcomes audit program. . . designed to ensure the reliability, clarity, and accuracy of the interpretation of mammograms"[4]; in practice, however, the audit legally required under the MQSA is limited.[7] The (voluntary) BMRAP also requires participating facilities to have a medical outcomes audit program.[6] The minimum audit requirements for ACR breast MR imaging accreditation are presented in **Box 1**.

Performing a more extensive audit, however, can be a powerful tool for practices committed to providing high-quality breast MR imaging. To achieve what the ACR terms a "basic clinically relevant audit," facilities must collect and analyze more than the minimum required data.[8] The clinically relevant audit is one that can be used to critically evaluate and improve interpretive quality. Specifically, facilities and individual radiologists performing such an audit will be able to compare multiple performance metrics derived from it against accepted criteria or benchmarks to identify deficiencies and specific metrics to target for improvement.

Although breast MR imaging auditing should generally follow standards established for mammography, some notable differences exist. Because screening breast MR imaging and diagnostic breast MR imaging examinations are composed of the same set of images, a screening breast MR imaging is simultaneously a complete diagnostic examination; positive screening and positive diagnostic examinations, therefore, share the same definition.[8] This unique feature of breast MR imaging is why use of a BI-RADS category 3 assessment, strongly discouraged for screening mammograms, may be considered for a screening MR imaging examination. If follow-up imaging is recommended at less than the routine screening interval, however, it is counted as a positive examination in the audit.[8] Another consequence of this modality specific definition is that purely screening metrics like recall rate and positive predictive value 1 are not applicable to breast MR imaging. Except in the few instances where modality-specific considerations necessitate a different approach, breast MR imaging and mammography audits are governed by the same principles.

Screening and diagnostic examinations must be segregated into separate audits to make meaningful comparisons between observed outcomes and benchmarks. Diagnostic breast MR imaging is often performed for the following indications:

symptoms or clinical findings suggestive of breast cancer, evaluation of newly diagnosed breast cancer, evaluation of response to neoadjuvant chemotherapy, and follow-up prior MR imaging findings or after MR imaging–directed biopsy. In contrast, screening breast MR imaging is performed only on an asymptomatic woman to detect early, clinically unsuspected breast cancer.[8] The prevalence of breast cancer can be expected to vary substantially between diagnostic and screening populations. Cancer detection rates and positive predictive values have been reported to be lower for screening than diagnostic breast MR imaging examinations.[9,10] Since 2007, the American Cancer Society has recommended annual screening breast MR imaging as an adjunct to mammography for women at sufficiently elevated risk for developing breast cancer[11] (Box 2). The American Cancer Society recommends against MR imaging screening for women of average risk (<15%), and neither recommends nor recommends against MR imaging screening for women at moderate risk (15%–20%). If moderate-risk or average-risk women are screened with breast MR imaging, practices may need to further stratify their screening breast MR imaging examinations by risk profile to determine whether minimum performance criteria are being met.

Performance Metrics

The ACR National Mammography Database and Breast Cancer Surveillance Consortium provide large volume benchmark data for screening and diagnostic mammography.[12–16] In the absence of any comparable breast MR imaging databases, however, similarly robust data are currently lacking for the modality. For the first time, the fifth edition of the *ACR BI-RADS Atlas* contains screening breast MR imaging benchmarks derived from 5 prospective trials in women with hereditary breast cancer risk[8,17–21] (**Table 4**). Whether the benchmarks are equally applicable to both expert and community practices remains to be seen. Other factors, such as practice volume and patient population (especially for practices that perform screening breast MR imaging on women of average risk for breast cancer), have the potential to affect generalizability of the benchmarks. To date, only a handful of practices have published screening MR imaging outcomes data evaluated against the ACR breast MR imaging screening benchmarks[9,10,22,23] (**Table 5**). Among these, there is some indication that the benchmarks are applicable to screening MR imaging in women with other high-risk profiles, including family history of breast cancer, personal history of breast cancer, history of chest irradiation, prior biopsy with atypia, or LCIS.[22]

Citing a lack of rigorous scientific data, the current *ACR BI-RADS Atlas* does not contain benchmarks for diagnostic breast MR imaging.[8] The task of identifying diagnostic performance benchmarks is almost certainly made more challenging by the variety of clinical scenarios in which diagnostic examinations are performed. Abnormal interpretation rates and other metrics may vary significantly with the clinical indication for the examination.[23] Subcategorization of diagnostic examinations may ultimately provide more granular insight into what constitutes acceptable performance for diagnostic breast MR imaging.

Table 4
Analysis of medical audit data: breast MR imaging screening benchmarks

Cancer detection rate (per 1000 examinations)	20–30
Median size of invasive cancers (in mm)	TBD
Percentage node-negative invasive cancers	>80%
Percentage minimal cancer	>50%
Percentage stage 0 or 1 cancer	TBD
PPV2 (recommendation for tissue diagnosis)	15%
PPV3 (biopsy performed)	20%–50%
Sensitivity (if measurable)	>80%
Specificity (if measurable)	85%–90%

From the ACR BI-RADS® Atlas, fifth edition; reprinted by permission of the American College of Radiology. All rights reserved. The most current version of the ACR BI-RADS® Atlas can be found at http://www.acr.org/Quality-Safety/Resources/BIRADS.

Although accreditation and the accompanying requirements of an audit are designed to address quality assurance, successful accreditation also has implications for reimbursement. Breast MR imaging is an advanced diagnostic imaging service and thus falls under the Medicare Improvement for Patients and Providers Act of 2008 (MIPPA). According to MIPPA, facilities billing for services under the technical component of part B of the Medicare Physician Fee Schedule must be accredited by a Centers for Medicare & Medicaid Services designated organization to qualify for Medicare reimbursement.[24]

ECONOMIC CONSIDERATIONS

The cost of breast MR imaging in the United States is frequently estimated in the literature to be 10 times higher than mammography,[25] costing approximately $1000 dollars per examination compared with $100 for mammography.[26–30] The cost of breast MR imaging is also higher than whole breast ultrasound and other emerging breast imaging technologies, such as molecular breast imaging (MBI).[31,32] Common uses of breast MR imaging include supplemental screening for women at high risk of breast cancer (>20% lifetime risk) as well as diagnostic evaluation of breast cancer and implant integrity.[11,28,33,34] Its widespread use and availability are limited, however, by its high cost and concerns regarding low specificity.[25] Beyond issues of reimbursement, other important economic considerations for the practice of breast MR imaging include cost-effectiveness, emerging competition from lower cost breast-imaging modalities, and the impact of price transparency.

Cost-Effectiveness of Screening

Image-based screening requires a defined group of patients for which benefit from screening has been demonstrated, minimal risk from both screening and downstream interventions, minimal development of interval cancers, and cost-effectiveness. Screening breast MR imaging cost-effectiveness models may be based on Medicare reimbursement, private insurance reimbursement, and/or billed charges from hospitals and imaging practices. Medicare reimbursement rates are frequently used, because Medicare data are readily available and demonstrate less variation compared with private insurer reimbursement. Incorporating any of these sources alone into cost-effectiveness models may, however, poorly reflect actual costs for a given individual or society. For example, breast MR imaging screening studies based on Medicare reimbursement are

Table 5
Screening Breast MR Outcomes

	Screening Benchmark	Niell et al,[10] 2014	Lee et al,[23] 2014	Chikarmane et al,[9] 2017	Strigel et al,[22] 2017
Number of examinations	—	1313	3989	3297	860
Number of lesion assessments	—	—	—	5927	—
Abnormal interpretation rate	—	—	—	—	—
BI-RADS 3 considered positive	—	12%	21%	9.3%	15.6%
BI-RADS 3 considered negative	—	6%	11%	NR	10.6%
Cancer detection rate (per 1000)	20–30	14	NR	16.7	22.1
PPV2 (biopsy recommended)	15%	24.0%	NR	22.9%	21.6%
PPV3 (biopsy performed)	20%–50%	27.0%	NR	27.0%	23.8%

Abbreviation: NR, not reported.

likely to underestimate the costs of screening in a population of young BRCA1 or BRCA2 carriers not eligible for Medicare[35,36]; large disparities may exist between Medicare and private insurers reimbursement rates.[37] Additionally, out-of-pocket expenses that have an impact on patient access to breast MR imaging vary depending on copay status[34] and annual deductibles and, therefore, are difficult to incorporate into cost-effectiveness models. Estimating costs from hospital billing statements is also problematic, because total billed charges differ among facilities and likely overestimate actual reimbursement amounts.

Cost-effectiveness modeling also requires assumptions to be made that introduce uncertainty, such as the estimated benefit of early detection in terms of survival prolongation.[26,38] To be cost-effective, a screening examination must be cost neutral or less expensive than no screening at all or, alternatively, performed at an acceptable cost for the outcome procured.[28] Although no consensus exists, threshold levels of cost-effectiveness in the medical literature typically range from $50,000 to $100,000 dollars per quality-adjusted life-year saved.[27,28,35,39] Screening breast MR imaging meets this threshold of cost-effectiveness only for certain defined indications.[28,40]

Specifically, screening breast MR imaging is currently considered cost-effective for women at a greater than 20% lifetime risk of developing cancer.[27,28,41] This includes women with known BRCA1 or BRCA2 mutations[11,25–28,35,42–44] and women with a strong family history of cancer but no known genetic mutation.[27,28,35] Other groups in which it is cost-effective include women with a greater than 1% to 3% prevalence of breast cancer,[26,38] such as women between 10 years and 30 years of age who received chest irradiation.[11,41] Research also suggests that MR imaging surveillance after breast-conserving therapy may be cost-effective given MR imaging sensitivity for detecting recurrence compared with mammography.[33]

Cost-effective screening thus requires a satisfactory balance between imaging costs and the prevalence of treatable cancer in the population being screened. Despite being more sensitive than mammography, screening breast MR imaging is not currently cost-effective for average or intermediate risk women given the high expense of breast MR imaging.[25,26,40] If expenses associated with breast MR imaging could be lowered, however, then cost-effective supplemental MR imaging screening may eventually be feasible for these women as well.[25,38] Abbreviated breast MR imaging techniques that shorten imaging times to 10 minutes or less are being evaluated as one possible way to lower the cost of breast MR imaging for purposes of supplemental screening.[27,40,45]

Improved identification and screening of women at elevated risk of breast cancer could also facilitate more cost-effective supplemental breast MR imaging and may also improve clinical outcomes. Unfortunately, it can be difficult to identify women at high lifetime risk of breast cancer prior to diagnosis of a malignant or high-risk lesion in themselves or a family member.[38] The accuracy of current genetic risk models in predicting lifetime risk of breast cancer has also been questioned.[11,28,46] More refined and inclusive risk models, including those that address breast parenchymal density, may be necessary to identify women who will benefit maximally from supplemental MR imaging screening.[36,47] Finally, it is important to remember that MR imaging is the single most sensitive screening modality for breast cancer, regardless of risk. Similar to mammography, widespread availability could be beneficial to society if costs and risk of false positive results can be maintained at reasonably low levels.[25,38,48]

Competing Modalities

Mammography, ultrasound, and MR imaging have been the standard breast imaging modalities for more than a decade. Use of other modalities, such as contrast-enhanced digital mammography (CEDM) and MBI is increasing, however, often as an alternative to breast MR imaging for specific indications.

CEDM provides standard mammographic-type images in addition to contrast-enhanced subtracted images obtained after the intravenous administration of iodinated contrast. CEDM and MR imaging both evaluate lesion vascularity and early research suggests that the sensitivity of CEDM for breast cancer detection may approximate that of MR imaging.[49,50] Benefits of CEDM compared with MR imaging include lower cost of equipment acquisition (often requiring only a software upgrade to existing mammography units), lower cost of imaging (cost of CEDM is typically that of a diagnostic mammogram plus the cost of iodinated contrast material), reduced imaging time, reduced interpretation time, and improved patient comfort (ie, no claustrophobia).[49,51,52] Disadvantages of CEDM compared with MR imaging include exposure to low doses of ionizing radiation,[49] risk of adverse events from iodinated contrast materials, and inferior visualization of the entire axilla, chest wall, and internal mammary chain.

Current MBI produces superior resolution images from reduced doses of technetium Tc 99m sestamibi compared with prior-generation breast-specific gamma imaging systems. MBI systems now image at a 6.5 mCi to 8 mCi dose compared with 20 mCi to 30 mCi for breast specific gamma imaging, largely through using dual-head solid cadmium-zinc-telluride detectors. Potential advantages of MBI over MR imaging include lower cost of equipment acquisition, lower imaging costs (typically in the range of $300 to $500),[30,32] better patient tolerance of imaging (ie, no claustrophobia), avoidance of intravenous contrast media, and faster image interpretation time. Disadvantages include exposure to low doses of ionizing radiation, longer image acquisition times, and limited visualization of the entire axilla, chest wall, and internal mammary chains.

Neither CEDM nor MBI is likely to replace MR imaging as a reference-standard technique in breast imaging. CEDM and MBI may be performed, however, at less than half the cost of MR imaging while potentially offering many of the benefits of MR imaging. In terms of supplemental screening, automated breast ultrasound, digital breast tomosynthesis, and MBI have been studied as alternatives to MR imaging[30,32,53] (see **Table 6** for comparison of diagnostic performance and costs between these breast imaging modalities).

If payment models shift from fee-for-service models toward alternative value-based models, or if other economic incentives prioritize lower cost imaging alternatives (such as certain cost-sharing models),[54] then CEDM or MBI could become increasingly attractive alternatives to MR imaging. MR imaging using abbreviated protocols could also become prioritized if these protocols lead to lower costs. Future studies are needed to better understand the relative strengths and limitations of CEDM, MBI, and abbreviated MR imaging techniques; early trials comparing the modalities are ongoing at the time of publication.

Price Transparency

The relative lack of price transparency in health care is a source of frustration for patients, referring clinicians, and radiologists alike.[55] Medical price transparency Web sites publish imaging examination costs online, allowing patients to compare costs from various imaging practices in the same geographic location.[56–60] In theory, price transparency enhances informed decision making among patients and referring providers by permitting actual costs of procedures to be compared.[59,61]

High-cost outpatient imaging examinations like breast MR imaging are especially amenable to price comparison and may be particularly targeted on price transparency Web sites. Importantly, these Web sites typically obtain cost data from a variety of sources, including insurance claim submissions, charge master documents, and self-reported cash-pay costs from patients or imaging providers. Comparing these costs to one another can be misleading. For example, charge master costs may not reflect actual health care costs

Table 6
Comparison of costs and diagnostic performance of tomosynthesis, whole-breast ultrasound, molecular breast imaging, and breast MR imaging for supplemental screening

Examination	Additional Cancers Detected per 1000 Examinations[1,3]	Cost Per Examination[2–5]	Cost Per Additional Cancer Diagnosis	Number Recalled for Additional Testing per 1000 Examinations[3]
Tomosynthesis	2	$56–$100	$28,000–$50,000	18–30 fewer
Whole breast ultrasound	3	$110–$165	$36,700–$55,000	130 more
MBI	8	$300–$500	$37,500–$62,500	65 more
Breast MR imaging	11	$539–$1000	$49,000–$90,900	90 more

Cost comparison demonstrates the lowest potential cost of supplemental screening per additional cancer diagnosis is found with tomosynthesis and the highest potential cost from breast MR imaging. Note, however, the relatively low yield of breast cancers detected per 1000 examinations with tomosynthesis compared with MR imaging. MBI may be attractive from a cost standpoint compared with other supplemental screening modalities given the relatively low number of patients recalled per 1000 examinations compared with whole-breast ultrasound and MR imaging and the relatively high yield of additional cancers detected per 1000 screening examinations.
Data from Refs.[30,32,63,64]

based on negotiated insurance contracts.[62] If costs based on charge master documents are compared with cash pay costs from hospital-based or nonhospital-based imaging, the cash pay costs could appear substantially less expensive even though they are actually similar to final facility costs based on negotiated insurance rates.

Price transparency could also lower imaging costs by encouraging price competition.[61] Patients may compare imaging costs among providers, thereby stimulating cost competition that may ultimately lower imaging costs.[56,57,60,61] Regarding breast MR imaging, however, patients should consider not only the examination cost but also the diagnostic quality of imaging, the diagnostic proficiency of the interpreting radiologist, and the clinical abilities of the network of breast specialists of which the radiologist is a member. If imaging costs are published without regard to quality outcomes, patient volume could be shunted toward the lowest cost providers regardless of quality.[56,59] Both costs and quality outcomes must be transparent if informed decision making based on the value of imaging services is desired.[56,59]

SUMMARY

Accreditation through the ACR BMRAP is necessary to qualify for reimbursement from Medicare and many private insurers. The program provides facilities with peer review and feedback on image acquisition and clinical quality. Adherence to ACR QC and technical practice parameter guidelines for breast MR imaging and performance of a medical outcomes audit program will maintain high-quality imaging and facilitate accreditation. Economic factors that are likely to influence the practice of breast MR imaging include cost-effectiveness, increasing competition with lower cost breast-imaging modalities, and price transparency, all of which may ultimately lower the cost of MR imaging and allow for greater utilization.

REFERENCES

1. ACR. About-Us. Available at: https://www.acr.org/~/media/ACR/Documents/PDF/About-Us/ACR-Fact-Sheet_F2.pdf. Accessed May 23, 2017.
2. Ellerbroek NA, Brenner M, Hulick P, et al, American College of Radiology. Practice accreditation for radiation oncology: quality is reality. J Am Coll Radiol 2006;3(10):787–92.
3. Destouet JM, Bassett LW, Yaffe MJ, et al. The ACR's Mammography accreditation program: ten years of experience since MQSA. J Am Coll Radiol 2005;2(7):585–94.
4. Mammography Quality Standards Act, 42 U.S.C §263b; 21 C.F.R §90012(f). (1992, reauthorized in 2004).
5. Hendrick RE. High-quality breast MRI. Radiol Clin North Am 2014;52(3):547–62.
6. ACR. Breast magnetic resonance imaging (MRI) accreditation program requirments. Available at: http://www.acraccreditation.org/~/media/ACRAccreditation/Documents/Breast-MRI/Requirements.pdf. Accessed May 15, 2017.
7. Monsees BS. The mammography quality standards act. An overview of the regulations and guidance. Radiol Clin North Am 2000;38(4):759–72.
8. Sickles E, D'Orsi CJ. ACR BI-RADS® follow-up and outcome monitoring. In: ACR BI-RADS® atlas, breast

imaging reporting and data system. Reston (VA): American College of Radiology; 2013.

9. Chikarmane SA, Tai R, Meyer JE, et al. Prevalence and predictive value of BI-RADS 3, 4, and 5 lesions detected on breast mri: correlation with study indication. Acad Radiol 2017;24(4):435–41.

10. Niell BL, Gavenonis SC, Motazedi T, et al. Auditing a breast MRI practice: performance measures for screening and diagnostic breast MRI. J Am Coll Radiol 2014;11(9):883–9.

11. Saslow D, Boetes C, Burke W, et al. American Cancer Society guidelines for breast screening with MRI as an adjunct to mammography. CA Cancer J Clin 2007;57(2):75–89.

12. Lee CS, Bhargavan-Chatfield M, Burnside ES, et al. The national mammography database: preliminary data. AJR Am J Roentgenol 2016;206(4):883–90.

13. Sprague BL, Arao RF, Miglioretti DL, et al. National performance benchmarks for modern diagnostic digital mammography: update from the breast cancer surveillance consortium. Radiology 2017;283(1):59–69.

14. Lehman CD, Arao RF, Sprague BL, et al. National performance benchmarks for modern screening digital mammography: update from the breast cancer surveillance consortium. Radiology 2017;283(1):49–58.

15. Carney PA, Sickles EA, Monsees BS, et al. Identifying minimally acceptable interpretive performance criteria for screening mammography. Radiology 2010;255(2):354–61.

16. Carney PA, Parikh J, Sickles EA, et al. Diagnostic mammography: identifying minimally acceptable interpretive performance criteria. Radiology 2013;267(2):359–67.

17. Kriege M, Brekelmans CT, Boetes C, et al. Efficacy of MRI and mammography for breast-cancer screening in women with a familial or genetic predisposition. N Engl J Med 2004;351(5):427–37.

18. Warner E, Plewes DB, Hill KA, et al. Surveillance of BRCA1 and BRCA2 mutation carriers with magnetic resonance imaging, ultrasound, mammography, and clinical breast examination. JAMA 2004;292(11):1317–25.

19. Leach MO, Brindle KM, Evelhoch JL, et al. The assessment of antiangiogenic and antivascular therapies in early-stage clinical trials using magnetic resonance imaging: issues and recommendations. Br J Cancer 2005;92(9):1599–610.

20. Kuhl CK, Schrading S, Leutner CC, et al. Mammography, breast ultrasound, and magnetic resonance imaging for surveillance of women at high familial risk for breast cancer. J Clin Oncol 2005;23(33):8469–76.

21. Sardanelli F, Podo F. Breast MR imaging in women at high-risk of breast cancer. Is something changing in early breast cancer detection? Eur Radiol 2007;17(4):873–87.

22. Strigel RM, Rollenhagen J, Burnside ES, et al. Screening breast MRI outcomes in routine clinical practice: comparison to BI-RADS benchmarks. Acad Radiol 2017;24(4):411–7.

23. Lee CI, Ichikawa L, Rochelle MC, et al. Breast MRI BI-RADS assessments and abnormal interpretation rates by clinical indication in US community practices. Acad Radiol 2014;21(11):1370–6.

24. Centers for Medicare and Medicaid Services (CMS) HHS. Medicare and medicaid programs: revisions to deeming authority survey, certification, and enforcement procedures. Final rule. Fed Regist 2015;80(99):29795–840.

25. Moore SG, Shenoy PJ, Fanucchi L, et al. Cost-effectiveness of MRI compared to mammography for breast cancer screening in a high risk population. BMC Health Serv Res 2009;9:9.

26. Taneja C, Edelsberg J, Weycker D, et al. Cost effectiveness of breast cancer screening with contrast-enhanced MRI in high-risk women. J Am Coll Radiol 2009;6(3):171–9.

27. Feig S. Comparison of costs and benefits of breast cancer screening with mammography, ultrasonography, and MRI. Obstet Gynecol Clin North Am 2011;38(1):179–96, ix.

28. Feig S. Cost-effectiveness of mammography, MRI, and ultrasonography for breast cancer screening. Radiol Clin North Am 2010;48(5):879–91.

29. Abbey CK, Wu Y, Burnside ES, et al. A utility/cost analysis of breast cancer risk prediction algorithms. Proc SPIE Int Soc Opt Eng 2016;9787 [pii:97871J].

30. Berg WA. Nuclear breast imaging: clinical results and future directions. J Nucl Med 2016;57(Suppl 1):46S–52S.

31. DeMartini WB, Ichikawa L, Yankaskas BC, et al. Breast MRI in community practice: equipment and imaging techniques at facilities in the breast cancer surveillance consortium. J Am Coll Radiol 2010;7(11):878–84.

32. Hruska CB, Conners AL, Jones KN, et al. Diagnostic workup and costs of a single supplemental molecular breast imaging screen of mammographically dense breasts. AJR Am J Roentgenol 2015;204(6):1345–53.

33. Shah C, Ahlawat S, Khan A, et al. The role of MRI in the follow-up of women undergoing breast-conserving therapy. Am J Clin Oncol 2016;39(3):314–9.

34. Hayes LM, Frebault JS, Landercasper J, et al. Extra-mammary findings in diagnostic breast magnetic resonance imaging among patients with known breast cancer: incidence and cost analysis. Am J Surg 2016;212(6):1194–200.

35. Lee JM, McMahon PM, Kong CY, et al. Cost-effectiveness of breast MR imaging and screen-film

mammography for screening BRCA1 gene mutation carriers. Radiology 2010;254(3):793–800.

36. Ong MS, Mandl KD. National expenditure for false-positive mammograms and breast cancer overdiagnoses estimated at $4 billion a year. Health Aff (Millwood) 2015;34(4):576–83.

37. Harvey SC, Di Carlo PA, Lee B, et al. An abbreviated protocol for high-risk screening breast MRI saves time and resources. J Am Coll Radiol 2016;13(11S):R74–80.

38. Lebovic GS, Hollingsworth A, Feig SA. Risk assessment, screening and prevention of breast cancer: a look at cost-effectiveness. Breast 2010;19(4):260–7.

39. Hirth RA, Chernew ME, Miller E, et al. Willingness to pay for a quality-adjusted life year: in search of a standard. Med Decis Making 2000;20(3):332–42.

40. Chhor CM, Mercado CL. Abbreviated MRI protocols: wave of the future for breast cancer screening. AJR Am J Roentgenol 2017;208(2):284–9.

41. Warner E, Messersmith H, Causer P, et al. Systematic review: using magnetic resonance imaging to screen women at high risk for breast cancer. Ann Intern Med 2008;148(9):671–9.

42. Plevritis SK, Kurian AW, Sigal BM, et al. Cost-effectiveness of screening BRCA1/2 mutation carriers with breast magnetic resonance imaging. JAMA 2006;295(20):2374–84.

43. Griebsch I, Brown J, Boggis C, et al. Cost-effectiveness of screening with contrast enhanced magnetic resonance imaging vs X-ray mammography of women at a high familial risk of breast cancer. Br J Cancer 2006;95(7):801–10.

44. Saadatmand S, Tilanus-Linthorst MM, Rutgers EJ, et al. Cost-effectiveness of screening women with familial risk for breast cancer with magnetic resonance imaging. J Natl Cancer Inst 2013;105(17):1314–21.

45. Kuhl CK, Schrading S, Strobel K, et al. Abbreviated breast magnetic resonance imaging (MRI): first post-contrast subtracted images and maximum-intensity projection-a novel approach to breast cancer screening with MRI. J Clin Oncol 2014;32(22):2304–10.

46. Amir E, Evans DG, Shenton A, et al. Evaluation of breast cancer risk assessment packages in the family history evaluation and screening programme. J Med Genet 2003;40(11):807–14.

47. Schousboe JT, Kerlikowske K, Loh A, et al. Personalizing mammography by breast density and other risk factors for breast cancer: analysis of health benefits and cost-effectiveness. Ann Intern Med 2011;155(1):10–20.

48. Poplack SP, Carney PA, Weiss JE, et al. Screening mammography: costs and use of screening-related services. Radiology 2005;234(1):79–85.

49. Lewis TC, Pizzitola VJ, Giurescu ME, et al. Contrast-enhanced digital mammography: a single-institution experience of the first 208 cases. Breast J 2017;23(1):67–76.

50. Fallenberg EM, Dromain C, Diekmann F, et al. Contrast-enhanced spectral mammography versus MRI: initial results in the detection of breast cancer and assessment of tumour size. Eur Radiol 2014;24(1):256–64.

51. Phillips J, Miller MM, Mehta TS, et al. Contrast-enhanced spectral mammography (CESM) versus MRI in the high-risk screening setting: patient preferences and attitudes. Clin Imaging 2017;42:193–7.

52. Ali-Mucheru M, Pockaj B, Patel B, et al. Contrast-enhanced digital mammography in the surgical management of breast cancer. Ann Surg Oncol 2016;23(Suppl 5):649–55.

53. Mahoney MC, Newell MS. Screening MR imaging versus screening ultrasound: pros and cons. Magn Reson Imaging Clin N Am 2013;21(3):495–508.

54. Burwell SM. Setting value-based payment goals–HHS efforts to improve U.S. health care. N Engl J Med 2015;372(10):897–9.

55. Paul AB, Oklu R, Saini S, et al. How much is that head CT? Price transparency and variability in radiology. J Am Coll Radiol 2015;12(5):453–7.

56. Rosenkrantz AB, Doshi AM. Public transparency web sites for radiology practices: prevalence of price, clinical quality, and service quality information. Clin Imaging 2016;40(3):531–4.

57. Wu SJ, Sylwestrzak G, Shah C, et al. Price transparency for MRIs increased use of less costly providers and triggered provider competition. Health Aff (Millwood) 2014;33(8):1391–8.

58. Mehrotra A, Brannen T, Sinaiko AD. Use patterns of a state health care price transparency web site: what do patients shop for? Inquiry 2014;51 [pii: 0046958014561496].

59. Durand DJ, Narayan AK, Rybicki FJ, et al. The health care value transparency movement and its implications for radiology. J Am Coll Radiol 2015;12(1):51–8.

60. Sinaiko AD, Rosenthal MB. Examining a health care price transparency tool: who uses it, and how they shop for care. Health Aff (Millwood) 2016;35(4):662–70.

61. Sinaiko AD, Rosenthal MB. Increased price transparency in health care–challenges and potential effects. N Engl J Med 2011;364(10):891–4.

62. Liberman A, Rotarius T. The challenge of the hospital chargemaster. Health Care Manag (Frederick) 2014;33(1):1–3.

63. Rhodes DJ, Hruska CB, Conners AL, et al. Molecular breast imaging at reduced radiation dose for supplemental screening in mammographically dense breasts. AJR Am J Roentgenol 2015;204:241–51.

64. 2016 Medicare physician fee schedule. Available at: http://www.acr.org/Advocacy/Economics-Health-Policy/Medicare-Payment-Systems/MPFS/2016-Proposed-Rule. Accessed March 7, 2017.